BASIC FIRST AID
POCKET GUIDE

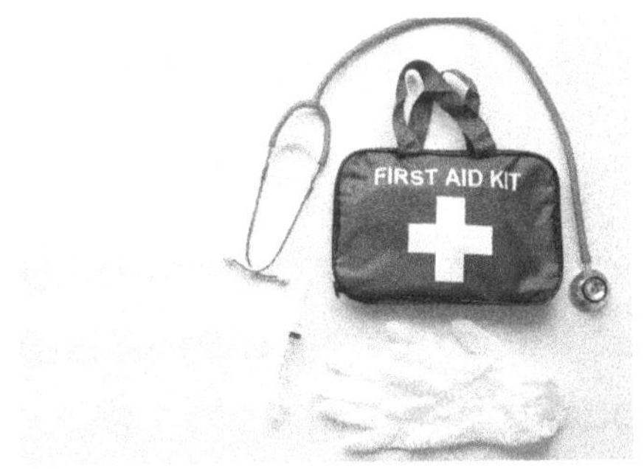

"Your Quick Reference Companion
for Handling Emergencies with
Confidence"

EMMA LYNCH

TABLE OF CONTENTS

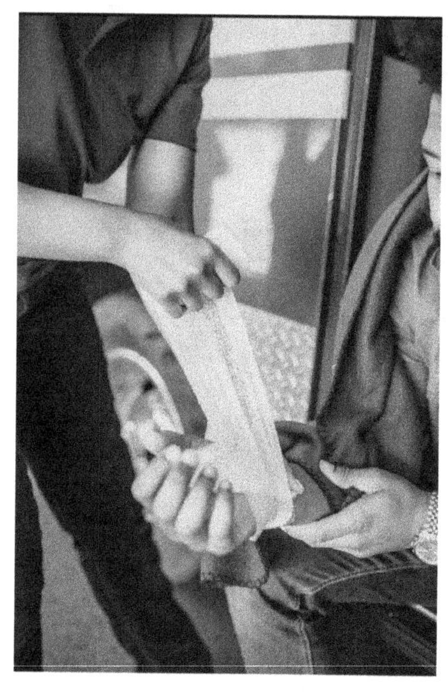

INTRODUCTION

In the realm of personal safety, a basic understanding of first aid can make the crucial difference between helplessness and empowerment. This Basic First Aid Pocket Guide serves as a compact and accessible companion for individuals seeking to navigate emergency situations with confidence and competence. In life's unexpected moments, whether at home, in the workplace, or out in the community, being equipped with fundamental first aid knowledge can be a lifeline.

This pocket guide is designed for quick reference, offering a concise overview of essential first aid principles and procedures. From understanding the ABCs of first aid – Airway, Breathing, Circulation – to mastering life-saving techniques such as Cardiopulmonary Resuscitation (CPR) and managing common injuries like cuts, burns, and fractures, this guide is a comprehensive resource tailored for everyday use. The importance of prompt and effective action cannot be overstated in emergencies, and this guide aims to empower individuals to take immediate, informed steps to aid those in need.

Whether you are a concerned parent, a diligent caregiver, or someone simply interested in fostering a safer environment, this Basic First Aid Pocket Guide equips you with the knowledge to respond effectively in critical situations. Compact in size but expansive in utility, it is a valuable tool for anyone committed to promoting well-being and preparedness in their community.

CHAPTER ONE

WHAT IS FIRST AID

First aid is the immediate and initial assistance or care given to someone who has been injured or is suddenly taken ill. Its key goals are to save lives, prevent the disease from worsening, and promote recovery. First aid can be administered by bystanders, trained laypeople, or healthcare professionals until more advanced medical help arrives.

Key components of first aid include assessing the situation, ensuring personal safety, calling for professional medical assistance, and providing basic care or interventions to the injured or ill person. Basic first aid techniques may include cardiopulmonary resuscitation (CPR), managing bleeding, immobilizing fractures, addressing burns, and supporting someone experiencing a medical emergency.

While first aid is not a substitute for professional medical treatment, it plays a crucial role in the chain of survival and can significantly improve outcomes in emergencies. Training in first aid equips individuals with the skills and knowledge needed to respond effectively to a variety of situations, from minor injuries to life-threatening incidents.

EMERGENCY RESPONSE

The Emergency Response section of the Basic First Aid Pocket Guide is a critical resource designed to equip individuals with the knowledge and skills needed to respond effectively in emergency situations. This comprehensive guide focuses on key aspects of emergency response, ensuring that users can assess and address crises with confidence.

ASSESSING THE SCENE

Assessing the scene is a fundamental component of effective emergency response, and it plays a pivotal role in ensuring the safety of both the rescuer and the victim. This crucial step is comprehensively addressed in the Basic First Aid Pocket Guide to equip individuals with the skills needed to make informed decisions in the midst of unexpected situations.

1. **Scene Safety:**
   - *Immediate Priority:* The guide underscores the immediate priority of ensuring the safety of everyone involved. Recognizing and mitigating potential hazards, such as fire, traffic, or unstable structures, is emphasized to prevent additional injuries.

   - *Personal Safety:* Users are reminded to prioritize their own safety before attempting to assist others, fostering a mindset that promotes effective and secure intervention.

2. **Victim Assessment:**
   - *Prioritizing Care:* Clear guidelines are provided on how to approach and assess the condition of the victim. This includes checking for responsiveness, breathing, and circulation, forming the foundation for subsequent first aid interventions.
   - *Severity Evaluation:* The guide educates users on assessing the severity of the situation, helping them determine the level of urgency and the appropriate actions to take.

3. **Calling for Help:**
   - *Timely Communication:* Recognizing the importance of professional medical assistance, the guide emphasizes the need for a prompt and clear emergency call. Details on what information to provide and how to communicate effectively with emergency services are outlined.

4. **Documentation:**
   - *Recording Details:* The guide encourages users to document relevant details about the scene and the victim, which can be valuable for healthcare professionals upon their arrival. This documentation may include the nature of the

incident, the number of individuals involved, and any observed injuries.

The detailed guidance on assessing the scene in the Basic First Aid Pocket Guide ensures that individuals approach emergency situations with a structured and informed mindset. By instilling the importance of scene safety, personal well-being, victim assessment, and timely communication, the guide empowers users to take decisive actions that can significantly impact the outcome of an emergency. This foundational knowledge is crucial for creating a safer environment and fostering a culture of preparedness among individuals in various settings.

CALLING FOR HELP

In the Basic First Aid Pocket Guide, the section on calling for help is a pivotal component of the emergency response protocol. It recognizes the critical role that professional medical assistance plays in ensuring the best possible outcome for the victim. The guide provides clear and concise instructions on the essential steps to take when reaching out for help during an emergency.

1. **Urgency of Professional Assistance:**
   - *Immediate Priority:* The guide emphasizes that calling for professional help is an immediate and top priority. This underscores the recognition

that certain emergencies require the expertise and resources of trained healthcare professionals.

   - *Collaborative Approach:* Users are encouraged to view their response as part of a collaborative effort with emergency services, reinforcing the importance of working together for a more effective outcome.

2. **Making an Emergency Call:**

   - *Maintaining Composure:* Recognizing the potential stress of the situation, the guide provides guidance on maintaining composure during the emergency call. This ensures that critical information is communicated clearly and efficiently.

   - *Information to Provide:* Clear instructions are given on the essential information to provide when making an emergency call. This includes details about the nature of the emergency, the number of individuals involved, and the location.

3. **Cooperating with Emergency Services:**

   - *Follow-up Instructions:* The guide emphasizes the importance of following any instructions given by the emergency dispatcher. This collaborative approach ensures that the information provided is effectively translated into the actions taken by professional responders.

   - *Continued Communication:* Users are encouraged to stay on the line until the dispatcher indicates it is appropriate to end the call. This ensures ongoing communication and allows for any additional information or instructions.

The Calling for Help section in the Basic First Aid
Pocket Guide serves as a practical and essential
resource for individuals faced with emergencies. By
highlighting the urgency of professional assistance,
providing guidance on making an emergency call,
and emphasizing collaboration with emergency
services, the guide contributes to a more effective
and coordinated emergency response. This
knowledge empowers individuals to take decisive
actions that can significantly impact the outcome of
an emergency situation.

ABCS OF FIRST AID (AIRWAY, BREATHING, CIRCULATION)

The ABCs of First Aid, detailed in the Basic First
Aid Pocket Guide, serve as the foundational
principles for immediate and life-saving
interventions. This essential section guides
individuals through a systematic approach to
assessing and addressing critical aspects of a
victim's condition during an emergency.

1. **Airway:**
   - *Clearing Obstructions:* The guide instructs
users on the crucial step of ensuring the victim's
airway is clear. Techniques such as the head
tilt-chin lift or jaw thrust are explained, allowing
users to effectively address any airway
obstructions.

- ***Recognition of Airway Issues:*** Clear
indicators of airway issues, such as abnormal
sounds or difficulty breathing, are highlighted. This
enables users to promptly identify and respond to
potential airway challenges.

2. **Breathing:**
  - ***Assessment of Breathing:*** The guide
provides a step-by-step process for assessing the
victim's breathing. This includes observing chest
movements, listening for breath sounds, and feeling
for breath on the rescuer's cheek.
  - ***Rescue Breathing Techniques:*** If the victim
is not breathing, the guide outlines rescue
breathing techniques, empowering users to deliver
effective breaths to support the individual's
respiratory function.

3. **Circulation:**
  - ***Checking for a Pulse:*** Users are guided on
how to check for the victim's pulse, a critical step in
assessing circulation. Locations for pulse checks,
such as the carotid or radial arteries, are
highlighted.
  - ***CPR Guidelines:*** The ABCs extend to the
initiation of Cardiopulmonary Resuscitation (CPR) if
no pulse is detected. The guide provides clear
instructions on chest compressions and the ratio of
compressions to rescue breaths.

4. **Integration of ABCs:**

- ***Systematic Approach:*** The guide emphasizes the importance of a systematic approach to the ABCs, recognizing that addressing airway, breathing, and circulation in a specific order is crucial for prioritizing interventions.

- ***Continuous Reassessment:*** Users are encouraged to continuously reassess the ABCs to adapt their interventions based on changes in the victim's condition.

The ABCs of First Aid section in the Basic First Aid Pocket Guide is a comprehensive resource that ensures users understand and can apply these foundational principles in emergency situations. By guiding individuals through the systematic assessment and intervention process, the guide empowers them to take immediate and informed actions that can make a significant impact on the outcome of a medical emergency.

CHAPTER TWO

CARDIOPULMONARY RESUSCITATION (CPR)

The Basic First Aid Pocket Guide dedicates a significant section to Cardiopulmonary Resuscitation (CPR), a critical and potentially life-saving technique for individuals experiencing cardiac arrest. This section provides detailed guidance on performing CPR for adults, children, and infants, ensuring that users are well-equipped to intervene in emergency situations.

ADULT CPR

Adult CPR, or Cardiopulmonary Resuscitation, is a life-saving technique designed to maintain blood circulation and oxygenation in individuals experiencing cardiac arrest. This critical intervention aims to increase the chances of survival until professional medical assistance arrives. The Adult CPR procedure, as outlined in the Basic First Aid Pocket Guide, involves several key steps:

1. **Recognition of Cardiac Arrest:**
   - *Signs:* The rescuer must recognize signs of cardiac arrest, such as unresponsiveness, absence of normal breathing, and the lack of a pulse. Quick

assessment and prompt identification are crucial for initiating CPR.

2. **Calling for Help:**
   - *Immediate Action:* Simultaneously with recognizing cardiac arrest, the rescuer should immediately call for professional medical assistance. This ensures that advanced care is on its way while CPR is initiated.

3. **Chest Compressions:**
   - *Proper Technique:* The guide details the correct technique for chest compressions. This includes placing the heel of the hand on the center of the chest (usually between the nipples) and using the upper body weight to compress the chest at least 2 inches deep for adults.
   - *Compression Rate:* The recommended compression rate is approximately 100-120 compressions per minute. This maintains effective blood circulation.

4. **Rescue Breaths:**
   - *Integration with Compressions:* While rescue breaths are traditionally part of CPR, the guide recognizes that untrained rescuers may be hesitant to provide them. In such cases, Hands-Only CPR, consisting only of chest compressions, is encouraged.
   - *If Trained:* For those trained in CPR, the guide provides instructions on delivering rescue

breaths, ensuring that each breath is effective in inflating the victim's lungs.

5. **Hands-Only CPR for the Untrained Rescuer:**

- *Simplified Approach:* Recognizing that not everyone may be trained in CPR, the guide introduces Hands-Only CPR. This technique involves continuous chest compressions without rescue breaths and is an accessible way for untrained bystanders to provide immediate assistance.

6. **Coordination with AED:**

- *Early Defibrillation:* The guide stresses the importance of coordinating CPR with the use of an Automated External Defibrillator (AED) if available. Early defibrillation can restore a normal heart rhythm.

7. **Continuous Reassessment:**

- *Adapting to Changes:* The rescuer is encouraged to continuously reassess the victim's condition and adapt interventions accordingly. This may involve adjusting compression depth, rate, or incorporating rescue breaths based on changes in the victim's responsiveness.

Adult CPR, as outlined in the Basic First Aid Pocket Guide, is designed to empower individuals to take immediate and effective action during a cardiac arrest emergency. By offering clear instructions and adaptable techniques, the guide aims to increase the likelihood of a positive outcome, contributing to the chain of survival in emergency situations.

CHILD CPR

Child CPR, or Cardiopulmonary Resuscitation, is a life-saving technique specifically designed for pediatric individuals experiencing cardiac arrest. The Basic First Aid Pocket Guide provides comprehensive guidance on Child CPR, recognizing the unique anatomical and physiological considerations for children. Here's an overview of the key steps:

1. **Recognition of Cardiac Arrest in Children:**
   - *Distinct Signs:* Rescuers are instructed to recognize signs of cardiac arrest in children, including unresponsiveness, the absence of normal breathing, and the lack of a pulse. Immediate recognition is critical for initiating Child CPR promptly.

2. **Calling for Help:**
   - *Simultaneous Action:* Similar to Adult CPR, calling for professional medical assistance is emphasized as a simultaneous action with recognizing cardiac arrest in children. Coordination with emergency services ensures a comprehensive approach to care.

3. **Adaptation of CPR Techniques for Children:**
   - *Compression Depth:* Child CPR involves adjusting the compression depth for children. Rescuers are guided to compress the chest at least one-third of the chest depth, typically around 2 inches, to maintain effective circulation.
   - *Compression Rate:* The recommended compression rate for Child CPR is approximately 100-120 compressions per minute, ensuring an appropriate balance between effectiveness and maintaining blood flow.

4. **Integration of Rescue Breaths:**
   - *Provision of Rescue Breaths:* Child CPR traditionally includes both chest compressions and rescue breaths. The guide provides instructions on delivering effective rescue breaths, highlighting the importance of proper technique and sufficient ventilation for pediatric patients.

5. **Hands-Only CPR for Untrained Rescuers:**
   - *Simplified Approach:* Recognizing that not all individuals may be trained in Child CPR, the guide introduces Hands-Only CPR for untrained rescuers. This approach involves continuous chest compressions without rescue breaths, offering a simplified yet effective method for immediate intervention.

6. **Coordination with AED:**

- *Early Defibrillation:* The guide emphasizes the importance of coordinating Child CPR with the use of an Automated External Defibrillator (AED) if available. Early defibrillation is crucial for restoring a normal heart rhythm in pediatric cardiac arrest cases.

7. **Continuous Reassessment:**
   - *Dynamic Response:* Rescuers are encouraged to continuously reassess the child's condition and adapt interventions accordingly. This includes adjusting compression depth, rate, or incorporating rescue breaths based on changes in the child's responsiveness.

Child CPR, as outlined in the Basic First Aid Pocket Guide, is tailored to meet the specific needs of pediatric patients during a cardiac arrest emergency. By providing clear instructions and emphasizing adaptability, the guide aims to empower individuals to take immediate and effective action, contributing to the chain of survival for children in emergency situations.

INFANT CPR

Infant CPR, or Cardiopulmonary Resuscitation, is a specialized life-saving technique crafted for infants experiencing cardiac arrest. The Basic First Aid Pocket Guide offers detailed guidance on Infant CPR, recognizing the unique anatomical and physiological considerations for the youngest individuals. Here's an in-depth look at the key steps:

1. **Recognition of Cardiac Arrest in Infants:**
   - *Distinct Signs:* The guide educates rescuers on recognizing signs of cardiac arrest in infants, emphasizing factors such as unresponsiveness, the absence of normal breathing, and the lack of a pulse. Immediate recognition is crucial for initiating Infant CPR promptly.

2. **Calling for Help:**
   - *Simultaneous Action:* Similar to other CPR protocols, calling for professional medical assistance is emphasized as a simultaneous action with recognizing cardiac arrest in infants. Coordinating with emergency services ensures a comprehensive and timely approach to care.

3. **Gentle Adaptation of CPR Techniques for Infants:**
   - *Gentle Chest Compressions:* Infant CPR involves adapting compression techniques to the delicate nature of an infant's chest. Rescuers are guided to use two fingers to compress the chest about 1.5 inches deep, ensuring effective circulation while minimizing the risk of injury.
   - *Compression Rate:* The recommended compression rate for Infant CPR is approximately 100-120 compressions per minute, maintaining an

appropriate balance for effective chest compressions.

4. **Integration of Rescue Breaths:**
   - *Gentle Provision of Rescue Breaths:* Infant CPR includes the provision of gentle rescue breaths, recognizing the unique needs of infants for effective ventilation. The guide provides specific instructions on the proper technique and ventilation requirements for infants.

5. **Hands-Only CPR for Untrained Rescuers:**
   - *Simplified Approach:* Recognizing that not all individuals may be trained in Infant CPR, the guide introduces a simplified approach. Untrained rescuers can perform Hands-Only CPR for infants, involving continuous chest compressions without rescue breaths, offering a straightforward yet effective method for immediate intervention.

6. **Coordination with AED:**
   - *Early Defibrillation:* The guide underscores the importance of coordinating Infant CPR with the use of an Automated External Defibrillator (AED) if available. Early defibrillation is crucial for restoring a normal heart rhythm in infant cardiac arrest cases.

7. **Continuous Reassessment:**
   - *Dynamic Response:* Rescuers are encouraged to continuously reassess the infant's condition and adapt interventions accordingly. This

includes adjusting compression depth, rate, or incorporating rescue breaths based on changes in the infant's responsiveness.

Infant CPR, as outlined in the Basic First Aid Pocket Guide, is characterized by its delicate and precise techniques to meet the specific needs of the youngest patients during a cardiac arrest emergency. By providing clear instructions and emphasizing adaptability, the guide aims to empower individuals to take immediate and effective action, contributing to the chain of survival for infants in emergency situations.

INTEGRATION WITH ABCS

The integration of CPR with the ABCs (Airway, Breathing, Circulation) is a foundational aspect emphasized in the Basic First Aid Pocket Guide. This coordinated approach ensures a systematic and comprehensive response to cardiac arrest situations, maintaining a focus on the critical elements of immediate care.

1. **Recognition of Cardiac Arrest and Airway Assessment:**
   - *Immediate Recognition:* The rescuer first recognizes signs of cardiac arrest, prompting the initiation of CPR. Simultaneously, attention is given to the victim's airway, ensuring it is clear of obstructions.

- *Adaptation for CPR:* The integration begins by recognizing that, during CPR, the airway remains a priority. Proper head positioning and airway assessment are part of the ongoing response.

2. **Calling for Help and Breathing Assessment:**

- *Simultaneous Actions:* While initiating CPR, the rescuer calls for professional medical assistance. Meanwhile, attention is given to assessing the victim's breathing, including rescue breaths in traditional CPR or Hands-Only CPR for untrained rescuers.

- *Adaptation for CPR:* The guide ensures that the coordination of calling for help and assessing breathing is seamlessly integrated with the CPR technique being employed.

3. **Chest Compressions and Circulation Assessment:**

- *Immediate Chest Compressions:* Chest compressions are initiated promptly, ensuring continuous blood circulation. The guide emphasizes proper compression technique and depth.

- *Adaptation for CPR:* As chest compressions are ongoing, the circulatory aspect of the ABCs is maintained. The rescuer continuously reassesses circulation through chest compressions.

4. **Integration with Rescue Breaths:**

- *Traditional CPR:* For those trained in CPR, rescue breaths are integrated into the sequence. The guide provides clear instructions on the ratio of compressions to rescue breaths.
- *Hands-Only CPR:* Untrained rescuers, opting for Hands-Only CPR, focus solely on chest compressions, aligning with the simplified approach while ensuring continued attention to airway, breathing, and circulation.

5. **Coordination with AED Use:**
   - *Introduction of AED:* The guide reinforces the coordination of CPR with the use of an Automated External Defibrillator (AED), emphasizing the importance of early defibrillation in restoring a normal heart rhythm.
   - *Integration with CPR:* Whether initiating chest compressions, rescue breaths, or using an AED, the ABCs remain integral to the overall response, reflecting a holistic approach to immediate care.

6. **Continuous Reassessment and Adaptation:**
   - *Dynamic Nature:* Throughout the CPR process, the rescuer is encouraged to continuously reassess the victim's condition. Adaptations to the intervention, including adjustments in compression depth, rate, or the incorporation of rescue breaths, are made based on changes in the victim's responsiveness.

The integration of CPR with the ABCs, as guided by the Basic First Aid Pocket Guide, ensures a synchronized and well-coordinated response to cardiac arrest emergencies. By maintaining a focus on airway, breathing, and circulation throughout the CPR sequence, the guide empowers individuals to deliver immediate and effective care, contributing to the overall chain of survival.

AED Use

The Basic First Aid Pocket Guide underscores the importance of Automated External Defibrillator (AED) use in cardiac arrest situations. AEDs are portable devices designed to deliver an electric shock to the heart, potentially restoring a normal rhythm during sudden cardiac arrest. Here's a breakdown of AED use as outlined in the guide:

1. **Recognition of Cardiac Arrest:**
   - *Immediate Recognition:* The AED use begins with the recognition of signs of cardiac arrest. AEDs are specifically employed in cases where the victim is unresponsive, not breathing normally, and lacks a pulse.

2. **Calling for Help and Retrieving the AED:**
   - *Simultaneous Actions:* While calling for professional medical assistance, the rescuer should also instruct someone to retrieve the AED if

available. Quick access to the AED is crucial for prompt intervention.

3. **AED Activation and Preparation:**
   - *Switching On the AED:* The guide provides clear instructions on switching on the AED. Activating the device initiates voice prompts and visual cues to guide the rescuer through the steps.
   - *Pad Placement:* The rescuer is guided on proper pad placement, typically with one pad on the upper right chest and the other on the lower left side of the chest. The guide ensures precise placement for effective shock delivery.

4. **Clearing the Area and Analyzing the Heart Rhythm:**
   - *Ensuring Safety:* The guide emphasizes the importance of ensuring the victim and rescuers are clear of the area before the AED analyzes the heart rhythm.
   - *Automated Rhythm Analysis:* The AED automatically analyzes the victim's heart rhythm, determining whether a shock is advised. Voice prompts guide the rescuer through this process.

5. **Shock Delivery and CPR Resumption:**
   - *Clear Instructions for Shock Delivery:* If a shock is advised, the AED provides clear instructions for delivering the shock. Rescuers are encouraged to ensure that everyone is clear of the victim before pressing the shock button.

- *Prompt Resumption of CPR:* Immediately following shock delivery, the guide emphasizes the prompt resumption of CPR, starting with chest compressions.

6. **Continued AED Assistance:**
   - *Guidance for CPR Intervals:* The AED continues to guide the rescuer through CPR intervals, providing prompts for chest compressions and, if applicable, rescue breaths.
   - *Continuous Monitoring:* The guide reinforces the rescuer's role in continuously monitoring the victim's condition and adapting interventions based on the AED's guidance.

The integration of AED use in the Basic First Aid Pocket Guide highlights its role as a crucial component of the chain of survival. By providing clear instructions and emphasizing the coordination of AED use with CPR, the guide empowers individuals to effectively utilize this life-saving technology in emergency situations.

CHAPTER THREE

CHOKING

Choking occurs when a foreign object becomes lodged in the airway, obstructing the flow of air. This can lead to difficulty breathing and, if left unaddressed, may result in a life-threatening situation. Understanding how to respond to choking is crucial for providing immediate assistance. Here's an overview:

1. **Recognition of Choking:**
   - *Symptoms:* Choking victims may exhibit signs such as grasping their throat, inability to speak or breathe, and a distressed appearance. Promptly recognizing these symptoms is the first step in addressing a choking emergency.

2. **Assessment of Severity:**
   - *Observation:* Rescuers should assess the severity of choking by observing the victim's ability to cough or breathe. Severe choking is characterized by an inability to cough, speak, or breathe effectively.

3. **Immediate Action - Heimlich Maneuver (Abdominal Thrusts):**
   - *For Adults and Children:* Stand behind the victim, wrap your arms around their waist, make a

fist, and place it above the navel. Perform quick, upward thrusts to help dislodge the obstruction.
   - *For Infants:* Use a modified approach involving back blows and chest thrusts, considering the delicate nature of an infant's body.

4. **Continued Action Until Resolution:**
   - *Repeat Abdominal Thrusts:* Continue abdominal thrusts until the foreign object is expelled, or the victim can breathe and cough effectively. Encourage coughing between thrusts.

5. **Calling for Help If Necessary:**
   - *Professional Assistance:* If the choking persists, call for professional medical assistance. It's crucial to seek help while continuing efforts to relieve the obstruction.

6. **If Unsuccessful - CPR:**
   - *Transition to CPR if Unresponsive:* If the victim becomes unresponsive, initiate CPR. Chest compressions may help dislodge the object. If trained, provide rescue breaths as well.

7. **Continued Monitoring:**
   - *Vigilant Observation:* Monitor the victim's condition closely. If the obstruction is cleared, continue to reassure and monitor until professional medical help arrives.

Choking can happen unexpectedly, and a quick and informed response is essential. The Basic First Aid

Pocket Guide provides specific techniques, like the Heimlich maneuver, to address choking effectively. The key is to act promptly, assess the severity, and transition to additional measures like CPR if necessary, ensuring the best chance for a positive outcome in a choking emergency.

HEIMLICH MANEUVER FOR ADULTS

Performing the Heimlich maneuver on an adult is a critical skill for responding to choking emergencies. The Basic First Aid Pocket Guide outlines the following steps:

1. **Assess the Situation:**
   - Quickly determine how bad the choking is. If the person is unable to cough, speak, or breathe, immediate intervention is necessary.

2. **Position Yourself:**
   - Stand behind the choking adult and ensure both of your feet are firmly planted for stability.

3. **Place Your Arms:**
   - Wrap your arms around the adult's waist.

4. **Make a Fist:**
   - Form a fist with one hand, placing the thumb side against the middle of the adult's abdomen, just above the navel.

5. **Grasp with Other Hand:**
   - With your other hand, grab the fist.

6. **Perform Quick Abdominal Thrusts:**
   - Deliver quick, upward abdominal thrusts. Each thrust should be a distinct, separate movement.

7. **Continue Until Object is Expelled:**
   - Continue performing abdominal thrusts until the foreign object is expelled, and the person can breathe and cough effectively. Encourage the person to cough forcefully between thrusts.

8. **Seek Professional Medical Assistance:**
   - If the choking persists or if the person becomes unconscious, call for professional medical assistance immediately.

9. **CPR if Unresponsive:**
   - If the person becomes unresponsive, transition to CPR, starting with chest compressions. Check the mouth for visible obstructions before each set of compressions.

10. **Continuous Monitoring:**
   - Monitor the person's condition closely, adapting interventions as needed until professional help arrives.

Remember, the Heimlich maneuver is a technique to clear a blocked airway and should only be used when someone is truly choking. Always seek professional medical assistance if the choking persists or if the person becomes unresponsive. The Basic First Aid Pocket Guide provides these steps to empower individuals to respond effectively in adult choking emergencies.

BACK BLOWS AND CHEST THRUSTS FOR CHILDREN AND INFANTS

When responding to choking emergencies in children and infants, the Basic First Aid Pocket Guide recommends modified techniques, including back blows and chest thrusts. Here are the steps for each age group:

For Children (1 Year to Puberty):

1. **Assess the Severity:**
   - Quickly evaluate the severity of the choking. If the child is unable to cough, speak, or breathe effectively, intervention is crucial.

2. **Position Yourself:**
   - Position yourself behind the child and ensure both feet are stable.

3. **Deliver Back Blows:**
   - Use the heel of your hand to deliver five firm back blows between the child's shoulder blades. Each blow should be a separate and distinct movement.

4. **Check the Mouth:**
   - After back blows, check the child's mouth for any visible obstructions.

5. **Perform Chest Thrusts:**
   - If the obstruction persists, perform five chest thrusts. Place one hand on the center of the child's chest, just below the nipple line, and use quick, inward thrusts.

6. **Continue Until Object is Expelled:**
   - Alternate between back blows and chest thrusts until the foreign object is expelled, and the child can breathe and cough effectively.

7. **Seek Professional Medical Assistance:**
   - If the choking persists, call for professional medical assistance immediately.

8. **CPR if Unresponsive:**
   - If the child becomes unresponsive, initiate CPR, starting with chest compressions.

For Infants (Up to 1 Year):

1. **Assess the Severity:**
   - Quickly evaluate the severity of the choking. If the infant is unable to cough, cry, or breathe effectively, intervention is crucial.

2. **Position Yourself:**

- Position yourself behind the infant, supporting their head and neck with your hand.

3. **Deliver Back Blows:**
   - Apply five hard back strikes between the baby's shoulder blades with the heel of your hand. Each blow should be a separate and distinct movement.

4. **Check the Mouth:**
   - After back blows, check the infant's mouth for any visible obstructions.

5. **Perform Chest Thrusts:**
   - If the obstruction persists, perform five chest thrusts. Place two or three fingers on the infant's breastbone, just below the nipple line, and use quick, inward thrusts.

6. **Continue Until Object is Expelled:**
   - Alternate between back blows and chest thrusts until the foreign object is expelled, and the infant can breathe and cry effectively.

7. **Seek Professional Medical Assistance:**
   - If the choking persists, call for professional medical assistance immediately.

8. **CPR if Unresponsive:**
   - If the infant becomes unresponsive, initiate CPR, starting with chest compressions.

Always adapt techniques to the size and age of the child or infant. Seek professional medical help if the choking persists or if the child or infant becomes unresponsive. The Basic First Aid Pocket Guide provides these steps to empower individuals to respond effectively in choking emergencies involving children and infants.

CHAPTER FOUR

BLEEDING AND WOUND CARE

The Basic First Aid Pocket Guide emphasizes swift and effective actions when dealing with bleeding and wounds. Here's a detailed explanation of the key steps outlined in the guide:

1. **Assessment of the Situation:**
   - Quickly assess the severity of the bleeding and the nature of the wound. Determine if professional medical assistance is required based on the extent of the injury.

2. **Ensuring Safety:**
   - Prioritize safety for both yourself and the injured person. Utilize personal protective equipment, if available, to minimize the risk of infection.

3. **Control Bleeding:**
   - *Direct Pressure:* Apply direct pressure to the wound using a clean cloth, sterile bandage, or your gloved hand. This immediate action helps control bleeding and prevents further blood loss.
   - *Elevation:* If possible, elevate the injured area above the level of the heart. This aids in reducing blood flow to the wounded area, contributing to bleeding control.

4. **Wound Dressing:**

- ***Hand Hygiene:*** Wash your hands thoroughly before handling the wound to minimize the risk of infection.
- ***Cleaning the Wound:*** Gently clean the wound with mild soap and water. Avoid harsh substances like hydrogen peroxide, as they can be damaging to tissues.
- ***Antibiotic Ointment:*** Apply an antibiotic ointment to the wound to prevent infection.
- ***Sterile Covering:*** Use a sterile dressing or bandage to cover the wound. Ensure that it is applied snugly but not too tight to facilitate proper healing.

5. **Applying Pressure to Stop Bleeding:**

- ***Pressure Points:*** If direct pressure is insufficient to stop bleeding, apply pressure to the nearest pressure point between the bleeding site and the heart. This can further aid in controlling blood flow.

6. **Tourniquet (As a Last Resort):**

- ***Last-Resort Measure:*** In extreme cases where bleeding is severe and uncontrollable, a tourniquet may be considered as a last resort. Place it above the wound but not on a joint, and only use it when absolutely necessary.

7. **Seeking Professional Medical Assistance:**

- ***Determining Need:*** If bleeding persists, is severe, or the wound is deep and caused by a

serious injury, seek professional medical assistance
promptly.

8. **Continuous Monitoring:**
   - *Signs of Shock:* Monitor the injured person
for signs of shock, such as pale skin, rapid
breathing, or altered consciousness. Seek
immediate medical help if shock is suspected.

The Basic First Aid Pocket Guide provides these
detailed steps to empower individuals to respond
effectively in situations involving bleeding and
wounds. Remember, seeking professional medical
assistance is crucial for severe bleeding or deep
wounds.

CONTROLLING EXTERNAL BLEEDING

In the Basic First Aid Pocket Guide, controlling
external bleeding is a critical skill. Here are the
immediate steps to take when faced with external
bleeding:

1. **Assess the Situation:**
   - Quickly assess the severity of the bleeding and
the cause. Determine if professional medical
assistance is needed based on the extent of the
injury.

2. **Ensure Safety:**

- Prioritize the safety of both yourself and the injured person. Use personal protective equipment, if available, to minimize the risk of infection.

3. **Apply Direct Pressure:**
   - *Immediate Action:* Apply direct pressure to the wound using a clean cloth, sterile bandage, or your gloved hand. This helps control bleeding and minimizes blood loss.
   - *Firm and Continuous:* Maintain firm and continuous pressure on the wound. If the material becomes soaked with blood, do not remove it; instead, add more layers.

4. **Elevate the Injured Area:**
   - *Positioning:* If possible, elevate the injured area above the level of the heart. This helps reduce blood flow to the wounded area and aids in bleeding control.

5. **Pressure Points (If Needed):**
   - *Secondary Measure:* If direct pressure is insufficient, consider applying pressure to the nearest pressure point between the bleeding site and the heart. This can further assist in controlling blood flow.

6. **Tourniquet (As a Last Resort):**
   - *Limited Use:* In extreme cases where bleeding is severe and uncontrollable, a tourniquet may be considered as a last resort. Place it above

the wound but not on a joint, and only use it when absolutely necessary.

7. **Seek Professional Medical Assistance:**
   - *Prompt Action:* If bleeding persists, is severe, or the wound is deep and caused by a serious injury, seek professional medical assistance promptly.

8. **Continuous Monitoring:**
   - *Signs of Shock:* Monitor the injured person for signs of shock, such as pale skin, rapid breathing, or altered consciousness. Seek immediate medical help if shock is suspected.

Remember, the Basic First Aid Pocket Guide provides these immediate steps to empower individuals to respond effectively to external bleeding. Seeking professional medical assistance is crucial for severe bleeding or deep wounds.

DRESSING AND BANDAGING

In the Basic First Aid Pocket Guide, dressing and bandaging are crucial skills for wound care. Here's a step-by-step guide on how to dress and bandage a wound:

1. **Assess the Wound:**
   - Examine the wound to determine its size, depth, and severity. Decide if professional medical

assistance is required based on the nature of the injury.

2. **Ensure Safety:**

- Prioritize the safety of both yourself and the injured person. Use personal protective equipment, if available, to minimize the risk of infection.

3. **Clean Hands:**

- Wash your hands thoroughly before handling any dressing or bandage to prevent introducing bacteria to the wound.

4. **Clean the Wound:**

- Using a little soap and water, gently clean the wound. Avoid harsh substances like hydrogen peroxide, as they can be damaging to tissues.

5. **Apply Antibiotic Ointment:**

- If available, apply a thin layer of antibiotic ointment to the wound to prevent infection.

6. **Select the Appropriate Dressing:**

- Choose a sterile dressing that is appropriate for the size and type of the wound. Ensure the dressing covers the entire wound and extends beyond its edges.

7. **Secure the Dressing:**

- Use medical tape or adhesive strips to secure the edges of the dressing. Ensure it is snug but not too tight to allow for proper circulation.

8. **Apply Bandage:**

   - Choose an appropriate bandage based on the location and size of the wound. Start wrapping the bandage from the inner part of the wound outward, covering the dressing completely.

9. **Secure the Bandage:**

   - Use clips or adhesive strips to secure the ends of the bandage. Avoid wrapping too tightly to prevent compromising blood circulation.

10. **Check Circulation:**

   - Periodically check the circulation in the area beyond the bandage. Ensure the fingers or toes are warm, and the color is normal. Adjust the bandage if there are signs of impaired circulation.

11. **Seek Professional Medical Assistance:**

   - If the wound is deep, has embedded debris, or shows signs of infection, seek professional medical assistance promptly.

12. **Continuous Monitoring:**

   - Monitor the wound for signs of infection, such as increased redness, swelling, or discharge. Seek medical help if infection is suspected.

The Basic First Aid Pocket Guide provides these detailed steps to empower individuals to respond effectively when dressing and bandaging wounds.

Professional medical assistance is crucial for severe wounds or those requiring specialized care.

CHAPTER FIVE

BURNS AND SCALDS

Burns and scalds are injuries caused by exposure to heat, steam, hot liquids, or flames, resulting in damage to the skin and underlying tissues. Understanding the different degrees of burns is essential for providing appropriate first aid. Here's an overview:

1. **First-Degree Burns:**
   - *Characteristics:* burns that are superficial and only damage the skin's outermost layer.
   - *Symptoms:* Redness, pain, and mild swelling.
   - *First Aid:* Cool the burn under running cool (not cold) water for at least 10 minutes. Cover with a sterile dressing or clean cloth. Pain can be controlled using over-the-counter pain medications.

2. **Second-Degree Burns:**
   - *Characteristics:* Affect both the outer layer and part of the underlying layer of the skin.
   - *Symptoms:* Red, blistered skin, severe pain, and swelling.
   - *First Aid:* Cool the burn under running cool water for at least 10 minutes. Do not pop blisters. Cover with a sterile dressing. Seek professional medical assistance for extensive burns or burns on sensitive areas.

3. **Third-Degree Burns:**
   - *Characteristics:* Involve damage to the full thickness of the skin and underlying tissues.
   - *Symptoms:* Skin may appear white, brown, or charred. Nerve endings may be damaged, resulting in little or no pain.
   - *First Aid:* Do not attempt to cool the burn. Cover with a sterile, non-stick dressing. Seek emergency medical help immediately.

General Guidelines for Burns and Scalds:
- **Cooling the Burn:** For first-degree and minor second-degree burns, cool the burn under running cool water. Steer clear of ice or extremely cold water.
- **Avoiding Ice:** Ice can cause further damage to the skin. Use cool water instead.
- **Protecting from Infection:** Cover burns with a sterile dressing to protect from infection.
- **Pain Management:** Over-the-counter pain relievers can help manage pain for minor burns.
- **Seeking Medical Assistance:** For severe burns, burns on sensitive areas, or if there's uncertainty about the extent of the injury, seek professional medical assistance promptly.

Remember, burns and scalds require immediate attention, and the severity of the burn determines the appropriate first aid measures. Always prioritize safety and seek professional medical assistance for severe burns.

FIRST-DEGREE BURNS

First-degree burns are superficial injuries that affect only the outer layer of the skin. While they are less severe than second or third-degree burns, immediate care is crucial for relieving pain and promoting healing. Here's how to respond to first-degree burns:

1. **Assess the Situation:**
   - Quickly evaluate the burn to confirm it is a first-degree burn, characterized by redness and pain without blistering.

2. **Ensure Safety:**
   - Prioritize safety for yourself and the injured person. If it's safe to do so, remove the burn's source.

3. **Cooling the Burn:**
   - *Under Cool (Not Cold) Water:* Immediately cool the burned area under running cool (not cold) water for at least 10 minutes. This helps alleviate pain and prevents further tissue damage.

4. **Avoid Ice or Very Cold Water:**
   - *Caution:* Avoid using ice or very cold water, as it can exacerbate damage to the skin.

5. **Remove Tight Clothing or Jewelry:**

  - *Before Swelling Occurs:* Remove any tight clothing or jewelry near the burn site before swelling occurs.

6. **Covering with a Sterile Dressing:**
  - *Post-Cooling:* After cooling, cover the burn with a sterile, non-stick dressing or a clean cloth to protect it from infection.

7. **Pain Relief:**
  - *Over-the-Counter Medication:* If needed, over-the-counter pain relievers like ibuprofen or acetaminophen can be used to manage pain. Follow recommended dosage guidelines.

8. **Do Not Pop Blisters:**
  - *Caution:* If blisters form, do not pop them. Infection risk is increased when blisters are ruptured.

9. **Monitor for Infection:**
  - *Continuous Observation:* Keep a close eye on the burn for signs of infection, such as increased redness, swelling, or discharge. Seek medical help if infection is suspected.

10. **Seek Professional Medical Assistance If Necessary:**
  - *For Uncertain Cases:* If there's uncertainty about the severity of the burn or if the injured person has underlying health conditions, seeking professional medical assistance is advisable.

Always adapt first aid measures based on the individual's specific circumstances. The Basic First Aid Pocket Guide provides these immediate steps to empower individuals to respond effectively to first-degree burns.

SECOND-DEGREE BURNS

Second-degree burns are more severe than first-degree burns, affecting both the outer layer and part of the underlying layer of the skin. Here's how to respond to second-degree burns:

1. **Assess the Severity:**
   - Quickly assess the burn to confirm it is a second-degree burn, characterized by redness, blistering, and severe pain.

2. **Ensure Safety:**
   - Prioritize safety for yourself and the injured person. Remove the source of the burn if it's safe to do so.

3. **Cooling the Burn:**
   - *Under Cool (Not Cold) Water:* Immediately cool the burned area under running cool (not cold) water for at least 10 minutes. This helps alleviate pain and prevents further tissue damage.

4. **Avoid Ice or Very Cold Water:**

- *Caution:* Avoid using ice or very cold water, as it can exacerbate damage to the skin.

5. **Remove Tight Clothing or Jewelry:**
   - *Before Swelling Occurs:* Remove any tight clothing or jewelry near the burn site before swelling occurs.

6. **Covering with a Sterile Dressing:**
   - *Post-Cooling:* After cooling, cover the burn with a sterile, non-stick dressing or a clean cloth to protect it from infection.

7. **Pain Relief:**
   - *Over-the-Counter Medication:* If needed, over-the-counter pain relievers like ibuprofen or acetaminophen can be used to manage pain. Follow recommended dosage guidelines.

8. **Do Not Pop Blisters:**
   - *Caution:* If blisters form, do not pop them. Popping blisters increases the risk of infection.

9. **Seek Professional Medical Assistance:**
   - *For Extensive Burns or Sensitive Areas:* If the burn covers a large area, affects sensitive areas (face, hands, feet, genitals, or major joints), or if there's uncertainty about the severity, seek professional medical assistance promptly.

10. **Monitor for Infection:**

- *Continuous Observation:* Keep a close eye on the burn for signs of infection, such as increased redness, swelling, or discharge. Seek medical help if infection is suspected.

Always adapt first aid measures based on the individual's specific circumstances. The Basic First Aid Pocket Guide provides these immediate steps to empower individuals to respond effectively to second-degree burns.

THIRD-DEGREE BURNS

Third-degree burns are severe injuries that penetrate through the full thickness of the skin and affect underlying tissues. Responding promptly and seeking professional medical assistance is crucial. Here's how to address third-degree burns:

1. **Assess the Severity:**
   - Quickly assess the burn to confirm it is a third-degree burn, characterized by charred or white skin and potential numbness.

2. **Ensure Safety:**
   - Prioritize safety for yourself and the injured person. If it's safe to do so, remove the burn's source.

3. **Do Not Cool the Burn:**

- *Caution:* Unlike first and second-degree burns, do not attempt to cool a third-degree burn. Cooling can lead to hypothermia.

4. **Cover with Sterile Dressing:**
   - *Protection:* Cover the burn with a sterile, non-stick dressing or a clean cloth. Avoid applying adhesive bandages direct on the burn.

5. **Seek Professional Medical Assistance Immediately:**
   - *Urgent Action:* Third-degree burns require immediate medical attention. Make an emergency call or head to the closest hospital. Do not delay seeking professional help.

6. **Do Not Pop Blisters:**
   - *Caution:* If blisters form, do not pop them. Infection risk is increased when blisters are ruptured.

7. **Monitor for Shock:**
   - *Watch for Signs:* Monitor the injured person for signs of shock, such as pale skin, rapid breathing, or altered consciousness. Seek immediate medical help if shock is suspected.

8. **Do Not Apply Ointments or Creams:**
   - *Caution:* Avoid applying creams, ointments, or home remedies to third-degree burns. These can interfere with medical assessment and treatment.

9. **Keep the Person Calm:**
   - *Emotional Support:* Provide reassurance and keep the person as calm as possible. The shock from severe burns can be emotionally distressing.

10. **Do Not Use Ice or Very Cold Water:**
    - *Caution:* Avoid using ice or very cold water, as it can exacerbate damage to the skin and increase the risk of hypothermia.

Remember, third-degree burns are medical emergencies, and professional medical assistance must be sought immediately. The Basic First Aid Pocket Guide emphasizes the urgency of seeking help for severe burns.

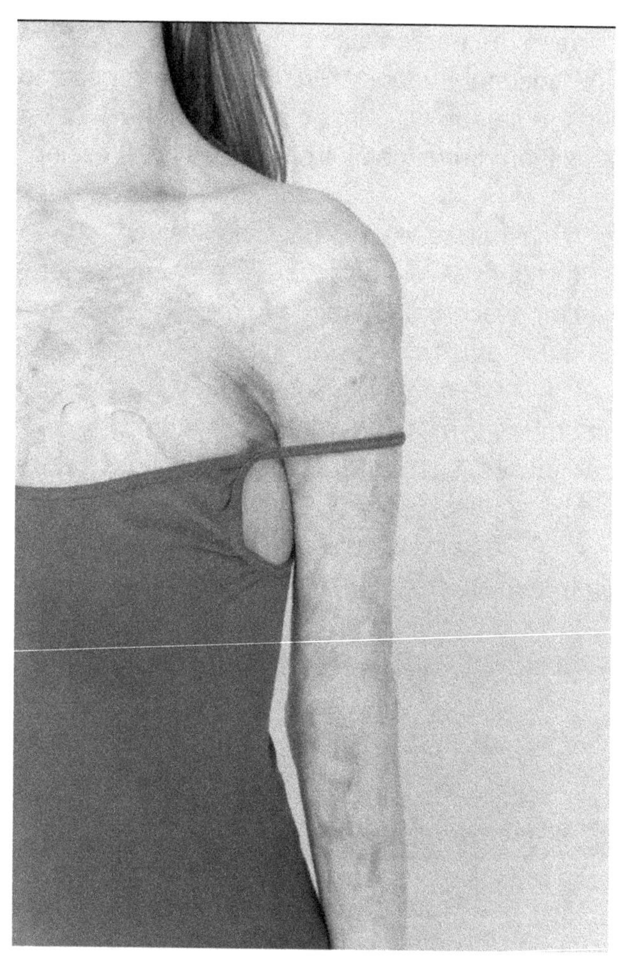

CHAPTER SIX

FRACTURES AND SPRAINS

Fractures and sprains are common musculoskeletal injuries that require prompt attention. The Basic First Aid Pocket Guide outlines the following steps to address fractures and sprains:

For Fractures:

1. **Assess the Situation:**
   - Quickly evaluate the injured area to determine if a fracture is suspected. Look for deformities, swelling, and pain.

2. **Ensure Safety:**
   - Prioritize safety for yourself and the injured person. Avoid moving the injured area unless there is an immediate threat to safety.

3. **Immobilize the Area:**
   - *Splinting:* If possible, immobilize the injured limb using a splint or by securing it to a stable object. This helps prevent further injury.

4. **Apply Cold Compress:**
   - *Pain and Swelling:* Apply a cold compress or ice pack wrapped in a cloth to the injured area to reduce pain and swelling.

5. **Seek Professional Medical Assistance:**
   - *Prompt Action:* Seek professional medical assistance promptly. Do not attempt to realign the bones or force the injured limb into a normal position.

6. **Keep the Person Calm:**
   - *Emotional Support:* Provide reassurance and keep the person as calm as possible. Immobilize the injured area and wait for professional medical help.

For Sprains:

1. **Assess the Severity:**
   - Quickly evaluate the injured area to determine if a sprain is suspected. Look for swelling, bruising, and pain.

2. **R.I.C.E. Method:**
   - *Rest:* Encourage the person to rest the injured area and avoid putting weight on it.
   - *Ice:* Apply a cold compress or ice pack wrapped in a cloth to the injured area for 15-20 minutes to reduce swelling.
   - *Compression:* Use a compression bandage to minimize swelling. A snug fit is ideal, but not too tight.
   - *Elevation:* Elevate the injured area above heart level to help reduce swelling.

3. **Seek Professional Medical Assistance:**

- *If Needed:* If the sprain is severe or if there is uncertainty about the injury, seek professional medical assistance.

4. **Immobilize and Support:**
   - *Using Splints or Bandages:* Immobilize and support the injured area using splints or bandages if necessary. Avoid putting unnecessary strain on the affected joint.

5. **Pain Relief:**
   - *Over-the-Counter Medication:* If needed, over-the-counter pain relievers like ibuprofen or acetaminophen can be used to manage pain. Follow recommended dosage guidelines.

Remember, the Basic First Aid Pocket Guide provides these immediate steps to empower individuals to respond effectively to fractures and sprains. Seeking professional medical assistance is crucial for proper diagnosis and treatment.

RECOGNIZING FRACTURES

Recognizing fractures promptly is crucial for providing appropriate first aid. Here are the key signs to look for and immediate responses outlined in the Basic First Aid Pocket Guide:

1. **Deformity:**

- *Sign:* Obvious deformity or misalignment of the injured limb or area.
   - *Immediate Response:* Avoid moving the injured area. Immobilize it using a splint or by securing it to a stable object. Seek professional medical assistance promptly.

2. **Pain:**
   - *Sign:* Severe pain, especially upon movement or touch.
   - *Immediate Response:* Encourage the person to remain still and avoid unnecessary movement. Apply a cold compress or ice pack wrapped in a cloth to the injured area to reduce pain and swelling.

3. **Swelling and Bruising:**
   - *Sign:* Swelling and bruising around the injured area.
   - *Immediate Response:* Apply a cold compress or ice pack wrapped in a cloth to the injured area for 15-20 minutes. Seek professional medical assistance.

4. **Limited Range of Motion:**
   - *Sign:* Difficulty or inability to move the injured limb or area.
   - *Immediate Response:* Immobilize the injured area using a splint or by securing it to a stable object. Avoid attempting to force the limb into a normal position. Seek professional medical assistance.

5. **Tenderness to Touch:**
   - *Sign:* Increased tenderness or pain upon touch.
   - *Immediate Response:* Minimize contact with the injured area. Immobilize it and seek professional medical assistance.

6. **Crepitus (Grating Sensation):**
   - *Sign:* Crepitus, a grating or crackling sensation during movement.
   - *Immediate Response:* Avoid movement of the injured area. Immobilize it using a splint or by securing it to a stable object. Seek professional medical assistance promptly.

7. **Guarding or Protecting the Injured Area:**
   - *Sign:* Instinctively protecting the injured area by holding it or avoiding movement.
   - *Immediate Response:* Encourage the person to keep the injured area still. Immobilize it and seek professional medical assistance.

Remember, early recognition of fractures is vital, and the Basic First Aid Pocket Guide provides these immediate steps to empower individuals to respond effectively. Seeking professional medical assistance is crucial for proper diagnosis and treatment of fractures.

IMMOBILIZING THE INJURY

When faced with an injury, especially fractures or suspected fractures, immobilizing the affected area is crucial to prevent further damage and alleviate pain. The Basic First Aid Pocket Guide outlines the following key steps for immobilizing injuries:

1. **Assess the Situation:**
   - Quickly evaluate the injured area to determine if immobilization is necessary. Look for signs of fractures, severe sprains, or any condition where movement may worsen the injury.

2. **Ensure Safety:**
   - Prioritize safety for yourself and the injured person. Avoid unnecessary movement and take precautions to prevent additional harm.

3. **Call for Professional Medical Assistance:**
   - If the injury involves fractures or if there's uncertainty about the severity, call for professional medical assistance promptly.

4. **Immobilize the Injured Area:**
   - *Splinting:* If possible, immobilize the injured limb using a splint. Ensure the splint extends beyond the joints above and below the injury.
   - *Stabilize with Support:* Use bandages or cloth to stabilize the injured area, avoiding unnecessary movement.

5. **Securing the Injury:**
   - *Ties or Bandages:* Secure the splint or support
with ties, bandages, or any available material.
Ensure the ties are snug but not too tight to avoid
cutting off circulation.

6. **Avoid Realignment Attempts:**
   - *Caution:* Do not attempt to realign bones or
force the injured limb into a normal position. This
should be done by medical professionals.

7. **Immobilize Joints:**
   - *Include Joints:* Immobilize joints both above
and below the injury to minimize movement and
prevent further harm.

8. **Comfort and Support:**
   - *Pillows or Cushions:* If the injury allows,
provide pillows or cushions around the injured area
for comfort and additional support.

9. **Stay Calm and Reassure:**
   - *Emotional Support:* Keep the injured person
calm and reassure them. Explain the steps you're
taking and the importance of seeking professional
medical assistance.

10. **Monitor for Shock:**
    - *Watch for Signs:* Monitor the injured person
for signs of shock, such as pale skin, rapid
breathing, or altered consciousness. Seek
immediate medical help if shock is suspected.

Remember, immobilizing the injury is a critical first aid measure, especially for fractures or suspected fractures. The Basic First Aid Pocket Guide provides these immediate steps to empower individuals to respond effectively while awaiting professional medical assistance.

R.I.C.E. METHOD FOR SPRAINS (REST, ICE, COMPRESSION, ELEVATION)

The R.I.C.E. method is a widely recognized approach for managing sprains to reduce pain, swelling, and promote healing. The Basic First Aid Pocket Guide outlines the following steps:

1. **Rest:**
   - *Encourage Rest:* Advise the person to rest the injured area and avoid putting weight on it. Minimizing movement helps prevent further injury.

2. **Ice:**
   - *Apply Cold Compress:* Immediately apply a cold compress or ice pack wrapped in a cloth to the injured area for 15-20 minutes. This helps reduce swelling and numbs the pain.
   - *Avoid Direct Contact:* Ensure the ice pack is not applied directly to the skin; use a cloth or towel as a barrier.

3. **Compression:**
   - *Use Compression Bandage:* Apply a compression bandage to the injured area to help control swelling. The bandage should be snug but not too tight to avoid interfering with circulation.
   - *Adjust as Needed:* Monitor the tightness of the compression bandage and adjust it if necessary to maintain comfort.

4. **Elevation:**
   - *Raise the Injured Area:* Elevate the injured area above the level of the heart whenever possible. This helps to reduce swelling by enabling fluids to drain away from the injury site.
   - *Support with Pillows:* Use pillows or cushions to support the elevated limb and provide comfort.

5. **Pain Relief:**
   - *Over-the-Counter Medication:* If needed, over-the-counter pain relievers like ibuprofen or acetaminophen can be used to manage pain. Follow recommended dosage guidelines.

6. **Seek Professional Medical Assistance:**
   - *For Severe Sprains:* If the sprain is severe, if there's uncertainty about the injury, or if symptoms persist, seek professional medical assistance.

7. **Avoid Putting Weight on the Sprained Area:**
   - *Limit Movement:* Encourage the person to avoid putting weight on the sprained area to prevent further strain.

8. **Monitor for Improvement:**
   - *Continuous Observation:* Monitor the injured person for signs of improvement. If there is no improvement or the condition worsens, seek medical help.

The R.I.C.E. method is an effective first aid measure for managing sprains, providing immediate relief, and facilitating the healing process. The Basic First Aid Pocket Guide emphasizes the importance of adapting these steps based on the specific circumstances and seeking professional medical assistance when needed.

CHAPTER SEVEN

HEAD INJURIES

Head injuries can range from mild to severe and require careful attention to minimize potential complications. The Basic First Aid Pocket Guide outlines the following information on head injuries:

Recognizing Head Injuries:

1. **External Signs:**
   - *Visible Injury:* Look for any visible injuries, cuts, or bruises on the head or face.
   - *Abnormalities:* Check for deformities or unusual bulges on the head.

2. **Symptoms:**
   - *Loss of Consciousness:* A person may lose consciousness or experience a brief blackout.
   - *Confusion:* Disorientation or confusion may be evident.
   - *Nausea and Vomiting:* Nausea and vomiting can occur after a head injury.
   - *Persistent Headache:* A persistent or worsening headache may be a sign of a more serious injury.
   - *Dizziness and Balance Issues:* Problems with balance or coordination may arise.

3. **Behavioral Changes:**

- *Mood Changes:* Notice any sudden changes in mood or behavior.
   - *Irritability:* Increased irritability can be a symptom.

Immediate Response to Head Injuries:

1. **Safety First:**
   - *Ensure Safety:* Prioritize safety for yourself and the injured person. Remove any immediate threats.

2. **Assess Consciousness:**
   - *Check Responsiveness:* Assess the person's level of consciousness. If unconscious, call for emergency medical assistance immediately.

3. **Stabilize the Head and Neck:**
   - *Minimize Movement:* If there's a risk of spinal injury, avoid unnecessary movement. Stabilize the head and neck.

4. **Control Bleeding:**
   - *Apply Pressure:* If there is bleeding from a wound, apply gentle pressure with a clean cloth or bandage.

5. **Seek Professional Medical Assistance:**
   - *Urgent Action:* Head injuries can be serious. Seek professional medical assistance promptly. Make an emergency call or visit the closest hospital.

6. **Monitor Vital Signs:**
   - *Continuous Monitoring:* Keep a close eye on the person's vital signs, including breathing and pulse. Perform CPR if necessary.

7. **Stay Calm and Reassure:**
   - *Emotional Support:* Keep the injured person calm and reassure them. Explain the steps being taken.

8. **Avoid Medications:**
   - *Caution:* Avoid giving medications unless directed by medical professionals.

Seek Medical Assistance for:

1. **Loss of Consciousness:**
   - *Even Brief:* If the person loses consciousness, seek immediate medical help.

2. **Severe Symptoms:**
   - *Severe Headache:* Persistent and severe headaches.
   - *Vomiting Repeatedly:* Persistent vomiting.
   - *Behavioral Changes:* Sudden and significant behavioral changes.

3. **Worsening Condition:**
   - *If Symptoms Worsen:* If symptoms worsen over time, seek medical assistance promptly.

Head injuries demand immediate attention due to the potential for serious consequences. The Basic First Aid Pocket Guide highlights the importance of swift and appropriate responses while emphasizing the need to involve professional medical assistance for thorough evaluation and treatment.

CONCUSSION AWARENESS

Concussions are a form of traumatic brain injury that require careful awareness, especially in situations where head injuries occur. The Basic First Aid Pocket Guide provides information on concussion awareness:

Recognizing Concussions:

1. **Common Signs:**
   - *Headache:* Persistent or worsening headache.
   - *Confusion:* Disorientation, confusion, or memory loss.
   - *Dizziness and Balance Issues:* Problems with balance or coordination.
   - *Nausea and Vomiting:* vomiting or nausea.
   - *Sensitivity to Light or Noise:* Increased sensitivity to light or noise.
   - *Changes in Sleep Patterns:* Disruption in normal sleep patterns.

2. **Behavioral Changes:**

- *Mood Swings:* Sudden changes in mood or behavior.
   - *Irritability:* Increased irritability.
   - *Difficulty Concentrating:* difficulty concentrating or concentration.

3. **Physical Symptoms:**
   - *Fatigue:* Persistent fatigue or lethargy.
   - *Blurred Vision:* Vision problems, including blurred vision.

Immediate Response to Suspected Concussions:

1. **Safety First:**
   - *Ensure Safety:* Prioritize safety for yourself and the injured person. Remove immediate threats.

2. **Assess Consciousness:**
   - *Check Responsiveness:* Assess the person's level of consciousness. If unconscious, call for emergency medical assistance immediately.

3. **Stabilize the Head and Neck:**
   - *Minimize Movement:* If there's a risk of spinal injury, avoid unnecessary movement. Stabilize the head and neck.

4. **Seek Professional Medical Assistance:**
   - *Urgent Action:* Concussions can have lasting effects. Seek professional medical assistance

promptly. Make an emergency call or visit the closest hospital.

5. **Monitor Vital Signs:**
   - *Continuous Monitoring:* Keep a close eye on the person's vital signs, including breathing and pulse. Perform CPR if necessary.

6. **Stay Calm and Reassure:**
   - *Emotional Support:* Keep the injured person calm and reassure them. Explain the steps being taken.

7. **Avoid Medications:**
   - *Caution:* Avoid giving medications unless directed by medical professionals.

Post-Injury Considerations:

1. **Rest and Recovery:**
   - *Physical and Cognitive Rest:* Encourage rest for both the body and mind. Limit activities that may worsen symptoms.

2. **Follow Medical Advice:**
   - *Professional Guidance:* Follow the guidance of medical professionals regarding recovery timelines and restrictions.

3. **Avoid Re-injury:**

- *Preventive Measures:* Take precautions to avoid re-injury. Avoid activities that may increase the risk of another head injury.

4. **Gradual Return to Activity:**
   - *Stepwise Approach:* Gradually reintroduce physical and cognitive activities under professional guidance.

Seek Medical Assistance If:

1. **Worsening Symptoms:**
   - *If Symptoms Worsen:* If symptoms worsen over time, seek medical assistance promptly.

2. **Persistent Issues:**
   - *If Symptoms Persist:* If symptoms persist, consult with healthcare professionals for further evaluation.

Concussion awareness is essential for timely and appropriate responses to head injuries. The Basic First Aid Pocket Guide emphasizes the importance of recognizing and responding to concussions promptly while highlighting the need for professional medical assistance for comprehensive evaluation and management.

SKULL FRACTURES

A skull fracture is a serious injury that demands careful attention and prompt medical assistance. The Basic First Aid Pocket Guide outlines the following steps for recognizing and responding to a suspected skull fracture:

Recognizing Skull Fractures:

1. **Visible Signs:**
   - *Open Wound:* A visible wound where the skull is broken or cracked.
   - *Deformity or Depression:* Noticeable deformity or depression in the skull.

2. **Symptoms:**
   - *Pain:* Intense pain at the site of the injury.
   - *Bleeding:* Bleeding from the nose, ears, or the site of the injury.
   - *Clear Fluid Drainage:* Clear fluid draining from the nose or ears may indicate cerebrospinal fluid leakage.
   - *Bruising or Swelling:* Bruising or swelling around the eyes or behind the ears.

3. **Behavioral Changes:**
   - *Altered Consciousness:* Loss of consciousness, confusion, or altered mental state.
   - *Seizures:* Seizures may occur after a skull fracture.

Immediate Response to Suspected Skull Fractures:

1. **Safety First:**
   - *Ensure Safety:* Prioritize safety for yourself and the injured person. Remove immediate threats.

2. **Assess Consciousness:**
   - *Check Responsiveness:* Assess the person's level of consciousness. If unconscious, call for emergency medical assistance immediately.

3. **Stabilize the Head and Neck:**
   - *Minimize Movement:* If there's a risk of spinal injury, avoid unnecessary movement. Stabilize the head and neck.

4. **Control Bleeding:**
   - *Apply Pressure:* If there is bleeding from a wound, apply gentle pressure with a clean cloth or bandage.

5. **Seek Professional Medical Assistance:**
   - *Urgent Action:* Skull fractures are serious. Seek professional medical assistance promptly. Call emergency services or go to the nearest hospital.

6. **Monitor Vital Signs:**
   - *Continuous Monitoring:* Keep a close eye on the person's vital signs, including breathing and pulse. Perform CPR if necessary.

7. **Stay Calm and Reassure:**
   - *Emotional Support:* Keep the injured person calm and reassure them. Explain the steps being taken.

8. **Avoid Medications:**
   - *Caution:* Avoid giving medications unless directed by medical professionals.

Post-Injury Considerations:

1. **Rest and Recovery:**
   - *Physical and Cognitive Rest:* Encourage rest for both the body and mind. Limit activities that may worsen symptoms.

2. **Follow Medical Advice:**
   - *Professional Guidance:* Follow the guidance of medical professionals regarding recovery timelines and restrictions.

3. **Avoid Re-injury:**
   - *Preventive Measures:* Take precautions to avoid re-injury. Avoid activities that may increase the risk of another head injury.

Seek Medical Assistance If:

1. **Worsening Symptoms:**
   - *If Symptoms Worsen:* If symptoms worsen over time, seek medical assistance promptly.

2. **Persistent Issues:**
   - *If Symptoms Persist:* If symptoms persist,
consult with healthcare professionals for further
evaluation.

Recognizing and responding to a suspected skull
fracture requires urgent action and professional
medical assistance. The Basic First Aid Pocket
Guide emphasizes the importance of swift and
appropriate responses while highlighting the need
for comprehensive evaluation and management by
healthcare professionals.

CARING FOR HEAD INJURIES

Caring for head injuries involves recognizing the
severity of the injury, providing immediate first aid,
and seeking professional medical assistance. The
Basic First Aid Pocket Guide outlines the following
steps:

Recognizing Head Injuries:

1. **Visible Signs:**
   - *Open Wounds or Cuts:* Assess for visible
wounds or cuts on the head or face.
   - *Deformities:* Look for deformities, unusual
bulges, or depressions on the skull.

2. **Symptoms:**

- *Loss of Consciousness:* Determine if the person has lost consciousness, even briefly.
   - *Confusion or Disorientation:* Check for confusion, disorientation, or memory loss.
   - *Nausea and Vomiting:* Observe for nausea and vomiting.
   - *Persistent Headache:* Note if there is a persistent or worsening headache.
   - *Dizziness and Balance Issues:* Look for problems with balance or coordination.

3. **Behavioral Changes:**
   - *Mood Changes:* Be aware of sudden changes in mood or behavior.
   - *Irritability:* Recognize increased irritability.
   - *Difficulty Concentrating:* Observe trouble focusing or concentrating.

4. **Physical Symptoms:**
   - *Fatigue:* Notice if there is persistent fatigue or lethargy.
   - *Blurred Vision:* Be attentive to vision problems, including blurred vision.

Immediate Response to Head Injuries:

1. **Safety First:**
   - *Ensure Safety:* Prioritize safety for yourself and the injured person. Remove immediate threats.

2. **Assess Consciousness:**

   - *Check Responsiveness:* Assess the person's level of consciousness. If unconscious, call for emergency medical assistance immediately.

3. **Stabilize the Head and Neck:**
   - *Minimize Movement:* If there's a risk of spinal injury, avoid unnecessary movement. Stabilize the head and neck.

4. **Control Bleeding:**
   - *Apply Pressure:* If there is bleeding from a wound, apply gentle pressure with a clean cloth or bandage.

5. **Seek Professional Medical Assistance:**
   - *Urgent Action:* Head injuries can be serious. Seek professional medical assistance promptly. Call emergency services or go to the nearest hospital.

6. **Monitor Vital Signs:**
   - *Continuous Monitoring:* Keep a close eye on the person's vital signs, including breathing and pulse. Perform CPR if necessary.

7. **Stay Calm and Reassure:**
   - *Emotional Support:* Keep the injured person calm and reassure them. Explain the steps being taken.

8. **Avoid Medications:**

- *Caution:* Avoid giving medications unless directed by medical professionals.

Post-Injury Considerations:

1. **Rest and Recovery:**
   - *Physical and Cognitive Rest:* Encourage rest for both the body and mind. Limit activities that may worsen symptoms.

2. **Follow Medical Advice:**
   - *Professional Guidance:* Follow the guidance of medical professionals regarding recovery timelines and restrictions.

3. **Avoid Re-injury:**
   - *Preventive Measures:* Take precautions to avoid re-injury. Avoid activities that may increase the risk of another head injury.

Seek Medical Assistance If:

1. **Worsening Symptoms:**
   - *If Symptoms Worsen:* If symptoms worsen over time, seek medical assistance promptly.

2. **Persistent Issues:**
   - *If Symptoms Persist:* If symptoms persist, consult with healthcare professionals for further evaluation.

Caring for head injuries requires a swift and appropriate response, along with seeking professional medical assistance for a thorough evaluation and management. The Basic First Aid Pocket Guide emphasizes the importance of recognizing and responding to head injuries promptly.

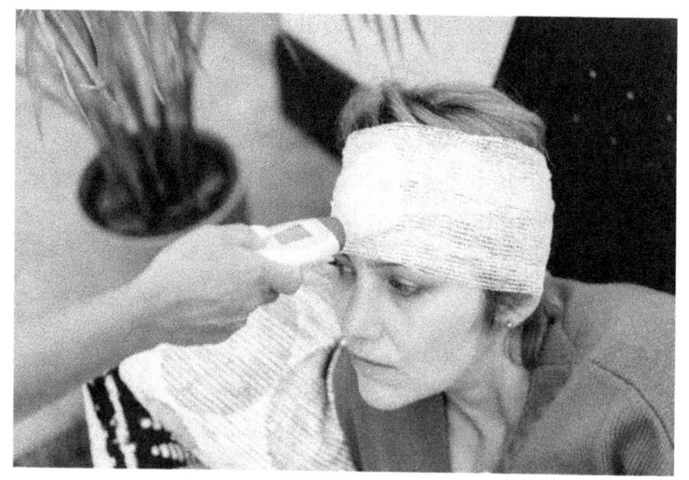

CHAPTER EIGHT

SEIZURES

Seizures can be frightening, but a calm and informed response is crucial. The Basic First Aid Pocket Guide outlines the following steps for recognizing and responding to seizures:

Recognizing Seizures:

1. **Uncontrolled Movements:**
   - *Jerking Movements:* Seizures often involve uncontrolled jerking movements of the limbs.
   - *Stiffness or Rigidity:* Some seizures may cause stiffness or rigidity in the body.

2. **Altered Consciousness:**
   - *Loss of Awareness:* The person may lose awareness of their surroundings.
   - *Unresponsiveness:* During the seizure, the person may not respond to stimuli.

3. **Involuntary Actions:**
   - *Involuntary Actions:* Seizures may lead to involuntary actions such as lip smacking or repetitive movements.

4. **Duration:**
   - *Varied Duration:* Seizures can vary in duration, from a few seconds to several minutes.

Immediate Response to Seizures:

1. **Safety First:**
   - *Ensure Safety:* Clear the area around the person of any sharp or dangerous objects. Create a safe space to prevent injury.

2. **Time the Seizure:**
   - *Note the Start Time:* Time the duration of the seizure. If the seizure lasts longer than 5 minutes, seek emergency medical assistance.

3. **Protect the Head:**
   - *Cushion the Head:* If possible, place a soft object or cushion under the person's head to protect it from injury.

4. **Do Not Restrain:**
   - *Avoid Restraining:* Do not restrain the person during the seizure. Let the seizure finish on its own.

5. **Turn to the Side:**
   - *Lateral Position:* Gently turn the person onto their side to help maintain an open airway and prevent choking.

6. **Do Not Put Anything in the Mouth:**
   - *Caution:* Do not attempt to force anything into the person's mouth. Contrary to common belief, placing objects in the mouth can cause harm.

7. **Stay Calm and Reassure:**
   - *Emotional Support:* Stay calm and reassure those around. Seizures can be frightening, but most seizures end on their own without lasting harm.

8. **After the Seizure:**
   - *Monitor Breathing:* After the seizure, monitor the person's breathing. If breathing is absent or irregular, begin CPR.

9. **Seek Professional Medical Assistance:**
   - *If Needed:* If it's the person's first seizure, lasts longer than 5 minutes, or if a second seizure follows immediately, seek professional medical assistance.

Post-Seizure Considerations:

1. **Recovery Position:**
   - *Recovery Position:* Once the seizure has ended, place the person in a recovery position on their side.

2. **Stay with the Person:**
   - *Monitor and Reassure:* Stay with the person and provide reassurance as they recover.

3. **Seek Medical Evaluation:**
   - *For First-Time Seizures:* If it's the person's first seizure, seek medical evaluation to determine the cause.

4. **Documentation:**
   - *Record Details:* If possible, document details of the seizure, such as duration and any observed symptoms, for medical professionals.

Remember, the Basic First Aid Pocket Guide provides these immediate steps to empower individuals to respond effectively to seizures. Seeking professional medical assistance for evaluation and guidance is essential, especially for first-time seizures or prolonged episodes.

IDENTIFYING SEIZURES

Identifying seizures involves recognizing various types of seizures, each presenting distinct characteristics. The Basic First Aid Pocket Guide outlines the primary types of seizures and their key features:

1. Generalized Tonic-Clonic Seizures (Grand Mal Seizures):

- **Description:** Involves both sides of the brain and typically has two phases.

  - *Tonic Phase:* Muscles stiffen, and the person loses consciousness.
  - *Clonic Phase:* Uncontrolled jerking movements occur.

2. Absence Seizures (Petit Mal Seizures):

- **Description:** Brief lapses in consciousness lasting a few seconds.

  - *Staring Episodes:* The person may appear to be staring into space.
  - *Brief Loss of Awareness:* Often mistaken for daydreaming.

3. Focal Onset Aware Seizures (Simple Partial Seizures):

- **Description:** Affects only one part of the brain without loss of consciousness.

  - *Altered Senses:* Changes in taste, smell, or touch.
  - *Involuntary Movements:* Simple repetitive movements.

4. Focal Onset Impaired Awareness Seizures (Complex Partial Seizures):

- **Description:** Alters awareness and may lead to confusion or unresponsiveness.

  - *Automatisms:* Repetitive behaviors like lip smacking or hand rubbing.
  - *Confusion:* Disorientation after the seizure.

5. Atonic Seizures (Drop Attacks):

- **Description:** Involves a sudden loss of muscle tone, leading to a person collapsing or falling.

  - *Abrupt Loss of Muscle Control:* Sudden and complete loss of muscle strength.

6. Myoclonic Seizures:

- **Description:** Involves brief, shock-like muscle jerks or twitches.

  - *Quick, Jerking Movements:* Usually occurs in the arms or legs.

7. Tonic Seizures:

- **Description:** Muscles suddenly stiffen, often causing falls.

  - *Stiffening Muscles:* Usually affects muscles in the back, arms, and legs.

Identifying Seizures: General Observations:

1. **Duration:**
   - *Short vs. Prolonged:* Note the duration of the seizure. Most seizures have a duration of a few seconds to several minutes.

2. **Motor Movements:**

- *Jerking, Stiffness, or Tremors:* Observe the type of motor movements, whether there's jerking, stiffness, tremors, or other involuntary actions.

3. **Consciousness:**
   - *Loss or Altered:* Determine if there's a loss of consciousness or altered awareness during the seizure.

4. **Postictal State:**
   - *After the Seizure:* Observe the person's state after the seizure (postictal state), which may include confusion or fatigue.

5. **Involuntary Behaviors:**
   - *Automatisms or Repetitive Actions:* Note any repetitive and involuntary behaviors that may occur during the seizure.

Recognizing these characteristics can help individuals differentiate between various types of seizures. However, it's essential to seek professional medical evaluation for a comprehensive diagnosis and appropriate management. The Basic First Aid Pocket Guide emphasizes the importance of understanding seizure types and responding effectively while awaiting professional medical assistance.

PROVIDING SUPPORT

Support for someone experiencing a seizure involves a calm and informed response to ensure their safety. The Basic First Aid Pocket Guide outlines the following steps to provide support during seizures:

1. Safety First:

- **Ensure a Safe Environment:**
  - *Remove Hazards:* Clear the area of any sharp or dangerous objects to prevent injury during the seizure.
  - *Create a Safe Space:* If possible, guide the person to a safe and open space.

2. Timing the Seizure:

- **Note the Start Time:**
  - *Time the Duration:* Start timing the seizure from the beginning. If the seizure lasts longer than 5 minutes, seek emergency medical assistance.

3. Protecting the Head:

- **Cushioning the Head:**
  - *Place a Soft Object:* If possible, place a soft object or cushion under the person's head to protect it from injury.

4. Do Not Restrain:

- **Allow the Seizure to Run Its Course:**
  - *Avoid Restraining:* Do not attempt to restrain the person during the seizure. Give the seizure time to pass.

5. Turn to the Side:

- **Maintaining an Open Airway:**
  - *Lateral Position:* Gently turn the person onto their side to help maintain an open airway and prevent choking.

6. Do Not Put Anything in the Mouth:

- **Caution:**
  - *Avoid Objects in the Mouth:* Do not attempt to force anything into the person's mouth. Placing objects in the mouth can cause harm.

7. Stay Calm and Reassure:

- **Provide Emotional Support:**
  - *Stay Calm:* Keep yourself calm, and reassure those around you. Seizures can be frightening, but most end on their own without lasting harm.

8. After the Seizure:

- **Monitoring Breathing:**

  - *Check Breathing:* After the seizure, monitor the person's breathing. If breathing is absent or irregular, begin CPR.

9. Seek Professional Medical Assistance:

- **If Needed:**
  - *Emergency Assistance:* If it's the person's first seizure, lasts longer than 5 minutes, or if a second seizure follows immediately, seek professional medical assistance.

Post-Seizure Considerations:

1. **Recovery Position:**

- **Positioning for Recovery:**
  - *Lateral Position:* Once the seizure has ended, place the person in a recovery position on their side.

2. **Stay with the Person:**

- **Monitor and Reassure:**
  - *Provide Reassurance:* Stay with the person and offer reassurance as they recover.

3. **Seek Medical Evaluation:**

- **For First-Time Seizures:**

  - *Professional Assessment:* If it's the person's first seizure, seek medical evaluation to determine the cause.

4. **Documentation:**

- **Record Details:**
  - *Note Observations:* If possible, document details of the seizure, such as duration and any observed symptoms, for medical professionals.

Remember, the Basic First Aid Pocket Guide provides these immediate steps to empower individuals to respond effectively to seizures. Seeking professional medical assistance for evaluation and guidance is essential, especially for first-time seizures or prolonged episodes.

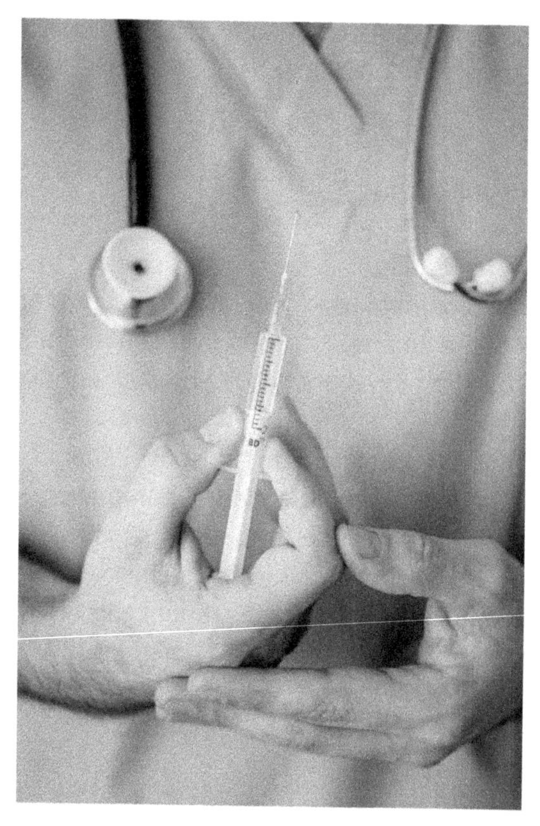

CHAPTER NINE

ALLERGIC REACTIONS

Allergic reactions can range from mild to severe, and a prompt response is crucial. The Basic First Aid Pocket Guide outlines the following steps for recognizing and responding to allergic reactions:

Recognizing Allergic Reactions:

1. **Mild Allergic Reaction:**
   - *Itchy or Watery Eyes:* Common symptoms include itching or watering of the eyes.
   - *Runny Nose:* Runny nose or congestion in the nose.
   - *Skin Irritation:* Mild skin reactions such as hives or itching.

2. **Moderate Allergic Reaction:**
   - *Swelling:* Swelling of the face, lips, or tongue.
   - *Difficulty Breathing:* Shortness of breath or wheezing.
   - *Abdominal Pain:* Abdominal discomfort or cramping.

3. **Severe Allergic Reaction (Anaphylaxis):**
   - *Difficulty Breathing:* Severe difficulty breathing or gasping for breath.
   - *Swelling of Throat:* Swelling of the throat or a feeling of a lump in the throat.

  - *Dizziness or Fainting:* Dizziness, lightheadedness, or loss of consciousness.
  - *Rapid Heartbeat:* A rapid or weak pulse.

Immediate Response to Allergic Reactions:

1. **Identify and Remove Allergen:**
  - *Identify Allergen:* If possible, identify and remove the allergen causing the reaction.
  - *Assist with Medication:* Help the person take any prescribed or over-the-counter allergy medication if available.

2. **Call for Professional Medical Assistance:**
  - *Urgent Action:* For moderate to severe reactions, call emergency services immediately. Anaphylaxis is a medical emergency.

3. **Administer Epinephrine (If Prescribed):**
  - *Inject Epinephrine:* If the person has an epinephrine auto-injector, assist them in using it. Follow the instructions on the device.
  - *Do Not Hesitate:* Do not hesitate to use epinephrine – it can be life-saving.

4. **Position for Comfort:**
  - *Comfortable Position:* Help the person sit or lie down in a comfortable position, whichever they prefer.

5. **Monitor Vital Signs:**

- *Continuous Monitoring:* Keep a close eye on the person's vital signs, including breathing and pulse. Be prepared to administer CPR if necessary.

6. **Stay with the Person:**
   - *Provide Support:* Stay with the person and provide reassurance until professional medical help arrives.

Post-Reaction Considerations:

1. **Monitor for Secondary Reactions:**
   - *Ongoing Monitoring:* Even after the initial reaction subsides, monitor for any secondary reactions. Anaphylaxis can sometimes have delayed or recurring symptoms.

2. **Seek Medical Follow-up:**
   - *Medical Evaluation:* Even after a mild reaction, it's advisable to seek medical follow-up to discuss and address potential triggers and preventive measures.

Remember, the Basic First Aid Pocket Guide provides these immediate steps to empower individuals to respond effectively to allergic reactions. Seeking professional medical assistance promptly is crucial, especially for severe reactions like anaphylaxis.

RECOGNIZING ANAPHYLAXIS

Anaphylaxis is a severe and potentially life-threatening allergic reaction that demands swift recognition and immediate action. The Basic First Aid Pocket Guide outlines key signs to recognize anaphylaxis:

Signs and Symptoms of Anaphylaxis:

1. **Respiratory Distress:**
   - *Difficulty Breathing:* Rapid onset of difficulty breathing or shortness of breath.
   - *Wheezing:* Audible wheezing or a high-pitched sound during breathing.

2. **Swelling:**
   - *Facial Swelling:* Swelling of the face, especially around the eyes and lips.
   - *Throat Swelling:* Swelling of the throat, leading to difficulty swallowing or a feeling of a lump in the throat.

3. **Circulatory Issues:**
   - *Drop in Blood Pressure:* A sudden drop in blood pressure leading to dizziness or fainting.
   - *Weak Pulse:* Weak or rapid pulse, indicating circulatory distress.

4. **Skin Reactions:**
   - *Hives:* Raised, red welts on the skin (hives) that may be itchy.

  - *Flushed or Pale Skin:* Skin may become flushed or pale.

5. **Gastrointestinal Symptoms:**
  - *Abdominal Pain:* Severe abdominal pain or cramping.
  - *Nausea and Vomiting:* Persistent nausea and vomiting.

6. **Mental Changes:**
  - *Confusion:* Mental confusion or a sudden change in consciousness.
  - *Feeling of Impending Doom:* A strong sense of impending doom.

Immediate Response to Anaphylaxis:

1. **Administer Epinephrine:**
  - *Inject Epinephrine:* If the person has an epinephrine auto-injector, help them use it immediately. Follow the instructions on the device.
  - *Do Not Hesitate:* Administer epinephrine promptly – it can be life-saving.

2. **Call Emergency Services:**
  - *Urgent Action:* Call emergency services immediately. Anaphylaxis is a medical emergency.

3. **Position for Comfort:**
  - *Comfortable Position:* Help the person sit or lie down in a comfortable position.

4. **Monitor Vital Signs:**
   - *Continuous Monitoring:* Keep a close eye on the person's vital signs, including breathing and pulse. Be prepared to perform CPR if necessary.

5. **Stay with the Person:**
   - *Provide Support:* Stay with the person and provide reassurance until professional medical help arrives.

Post-Reaction Considerations:

1. **Secondary Monitoring:**
   - *Ongoing Monitoring:* Even after the initial reaction subsides, monitor for any secondary reactions. Anaphylaxis can sometimes have delayed or recurring symptoms.

2. **Medical Follow-up:**
   - *Seek Urgent Medical Evaluation:* After an episode of anaphylaxis, seek urgent medical evaluation. The person may need additional treatment or guidance to prevent future occurrences.

Recognizing anaphylaxis involves being vigilant about the signs and acting promptly to administer epinephrine and call for professional medical assistance. The Basic First Aid Pocket Guide emphasizes the critical nature of these immediate steps to ensure the best possible outcome for someone experiencing anaphylaxis.

ADMINISTERING EPINEPHRINE (EPIPEN)

Anaphylaxis is a severe and potentially life-threatening allergic reaction that demands swift recognition and immediate action. The Basic First Aid Pocket Guide outlines key signs to recognize anaphylaxis:

Signs and Symptoms of Anaphylaxis:

1. **Respiratory Distress:**
   - *Difficulty Breathing:* Rapid onset of difficulty breathing or shortness of breath.
   - *Wheezing:* Audible wheezing or a high-pitched sound during breathing.

2. **Swelling:**
   - *Facial Swelling:* Swelling of the face, especially around the eyes and lips.
   - *Throat Swelling:* Swelling of the throat, leading to difficulty swallowing or a feeling of a lump in the throat.

3. **Circulatory Issues:**
   - *Drop in Blood Pressure:* A sudden drop in blood pressure leading to dizziness or fainting.
   - *Weak Pulse:* Weak or rapid pulse, indicating circulatory distress.

4. **Skin Reactions:**

- *Hives:* Raised, red welts on the skin (hives) that may be itchy.
  - *Flushed or Pale Skin:* Skin may become flushed or pale.

5. **Gastrointestinal Symptoms:**
  - *Abdominal Pain:* Severe abdominal pain or cramping.
  - *Nausea and Vomiting:* Persistent nausea and vomiting.

6. **Mental Changes:**
  - *Confusion:* Mental confusion or a sudden change in consciousness.
  - *Feeling of Impending Doom:* A strong sense of impending doom.

Immediate Response to Anaphylaxis:

1. **Administer Epinephrine:**
  - *Inject Epinephrine:* If the person has an epinephrine auto-injector, help them use it immediately. Follow the instructions on the device.
  - *Do Not Hesitate:* Administer epinephrine promptly – it can be life-saving.

2. **Call Emergency Services:**
  - *Urgent Action:* Call emergency services immediately. Anaphylaxis is a medical emergency.

3. **Position for Comfort:**

- *Comfortable Position:* Help the person sit or lie down in a comfortable position.

4. **Monitor Vital Signs:**
   - *Continuous Monitoring:* Keep a close eye on the person's vital signs, including breathing and pulse. Be prepared to perform CPR if necessary.

5. **Stay with the Person:**
   - *Provide Support:* Stay with the person and provide reassurance until professional medical help arrives.

Post-Reaction Considerations:

1. **Secondary Monitoring:**
   - *Ongoing Monitoring:* Even after the initial reaction subsides, monitor for any secondary reactions. Anaphylaxis can sometimes have delayed or recurring symptoms.

2. **Medical Follow-up:**
   - *Seek Urgent Medical Evaluation:* After an episode of anaphylaxis, seek urgent medical evaluation. The person may need additional treatment or guidance to prevent future occurrences.

Recognizing anaphylaxis involves being vigilant about the signs and acting promptly to administer epinephrine and call for professional medical assistance. The Basic First Aid Pocket Guide emphasizes the critical nature of these immediate steps to ensure the best possible outcome for someone experiencing anaphylaxis.

CHAPTER TEN

POISONING

Poisoning occurs when a person is exposed to harmful substances, either through ingestion, inhalation, or skin contact. These substances, known as poisons or toxins, can cause a range of adverse effects on the body. The Basic First Aid Pocket Guide provides an overview of poisoning, including common signs, immediate response, and post-incident considerations.

Common Signs of Poisoning:

1. **Ingestion:**
   - *Nausea and Vomiting:* Sudden onset of nausea or vomiting.
   - *Abdominal Pain:* Severe abdominal pain or cramping.
   - *Burning Sensation:* A burning sensation in the mouth, throat, or stomach.

2. **Inhalation:**
   - *Difficulty Breathing:* Rapid or difficulty breathing.
   - *Coughing or Choking:* Persistent coughing or choking.

3. **Skin Contact:**

- *Rashes or Burns:* Skin rashes, burns, or irritation at the contact site.

4. **General Symptoms:**
   - *Confusion:* Mental confusion or altered consciousness.
   - *Weakness or Dizziness:* Sudden weakness or dizziness.

Immediate Response to Poisoning:

1. **Call Emergency Services:**
   - *Urgent Action:* Call emergency services immediately. Provide information about the suspected poison and follow their guidance.

2. **Provide First Aid:**
   - *Do Not Wait:* If safe to do so, administer first aid based on the type of poisoning.
   - *Do Not Induce Vomiting:* Unless instructed by medical professionals, do not induce vomiting.

3. **Remove from Exposure:**
   - *Move to Fresh Air:* If the poisoning is due to inhalation, move the person to fresh air immediately.

4. **Administer Antidotes (If Available):**
   - *Follow Professional Guidance:* If antidotes are available and you are trained to use them, follow professional guidance.

5. **Perform CPR (If Necessary):**
   - *Start CPR:* CPR should be administered if the victim is not breathing and is unconscious. Follow the guidelines for adult, child, or infant CPR as appropriate.

6. **Save the Container:**
   - *Save the Poison Container:* If safe, save the container or any remaining substance to provide information to medical professionals.

7. **Stay with the Person:**
   - *Provide Support:* Stay with the person and provide reassurance until professional medical help arrives.

Post-Poisoning Considerations:

1. **Medical Follow-up:**
   - *Seek Urgent Medical Evaluation:* Even if initial symptoms subside, seek urgent medical evaluation to ensure comprehensive assessment and appropriate treatment.

2. **Reporting:**
   - *Provide Information:* Report the incident to relevant authorities if necessary.

3. **Preventive Measures:**
   - *Prevent Future Exposure:* Take measures to prevent future exposure to the toxic substance.

Recognizing and responding to poisoning requires swift action and professional medical assistance. The Basic First Aid Pocket Guide emphasizes the importance of calling emergency services immediately and providing necessary first aid while awaiting professional help.

INGESTED POISONING

Ingested poisoning occurs when harmful substances are swallowed. The Basic First Aid Pocket Guide outlines the following steps for recognizing and responding to ingested poisoning:

Recognizing Signs of Ingested Poisoning:

1. **Nausea and Vomiting:**
   - *Sudden Onset:* Rapid onset of nausea and vomiting.
   - *Repeated Vomiting:* Persistent and repeated episodes of vomiting.

2. **Abdominal Pain:**
   - *Severe Cramping:* Severe abdominal pain or cramping.
   - *Discomfort:* General discomfort in the abdominal region.

3. **Burning Sensation:**
   - *Mouth, Throat, or Stomach:* A burning sensation in the mouth, throat, or stomach.

   - *Painful Swallowing:* Difficulty swallowing due to pain.

4. **Dizziness or Weakness:**
   - *Sudden Weakness:* Sudden weakness or dizziness.
   - *Lightheadedness:* Feeling lightheaded or unsteady.

Immediate Response to Ingested Poisoning:

1. **Call Emergency Services:**
   - *Urgent Action:* Call emergency services immediately. Provide information about the suspected poison and follow their guidance.

2. **Do Not Wait:**
   - *Administer First Aid:* If safe to do so, administer first aid based on the type of poisoning.
   - *Do Not Induce Vomiting:* Unless instructed by medical professionals, do not induce vomiting.

3. **Save the Container:**
   - *Preserve Evidence:* If possible, save the container or any remaining substance for medical professionals to identify.

4. **Position for Comfort:**
   - *Comfortable Position:* Help the person sit or lie down in a comfortable position.

5. **Monitor Vital Signs:**

- *Continuous Monitoring:* Keep a close eye on the person's vital signs, including breathing and pulse. Be prepared to administer CPR if necessary.

6. **Stay with the Person:**
   - *Provide Reassurance:* Stay with the person and provide reassurance until professional medical help arrives.

Post-Ingested Poisoning Considerations:

1. **Medical Follow-up:**
   - *Seek Urgent Medical Evaluation:* Even if initial symptoms subside, seek urgent medical evaluation to ensure comprehensive assessment and appropriate treatment.

2. **Reporting:**
   - *Provide Information:* Report the incident to relevant authorities if necessary.

3. **Preventive Measures:**
   - *Prevent Future Exposure:* Take measures to prevent future exposure to the toxic substance.

In cases of ingested poisoning, a swift response is crucial. The Basic First Aid Pocket Guide underscores the importance of calling emergency services immediately, providing appropriate first aid, and seeking professional medical evaluation for comprehensive care.

INHALED POISONING

Inhaled poisoning occurs when harmful substances are breathed in. The Basic First Aid Pocket Guide outlines the following steps for recognizing and responding to inhaled poisoning:

Recognizing Signs of Inhaled Poisoning:

1. **Difficulty Breathing:**
   - *Rapid or Shallow Breaths:* Breathing becomes rapid or shallow.
   - *Labored Breathing:* The person may struggle to breathe or gasp for air.

2. **Coughing or Choking:**
   - *Persistent Coughing:* Continuous coughing spells.
   - *Choking Sensation:* A feeling of choking or tightness in the chest.

3. **Nausea or Vomiting:**
   - *Nausea:* Sudden onset of nausea.
   - *Vomiting:* May accompany nausea, depending on the substance inhaled.

4. **Dizziness or Weakness:**
   - *Sudden Weakness:* Sudden weakness or lightheadedness.
   - *Loss of Coordination:* Difficulty maintaining balance or coordination.

5. **Skin Irritation:**
   - *Rashes or Burns:* Skin irritation, burns, or redness around the nose and mouth.

Immediate Response to Inhaled Poisoning:

1. **Call Emergency Services:**
   - *Urgent Action:* Call emergency services immediately. Provide information about the suspected poison and follow their guidance.

2. **Move to Fresh Air:**
   - *Remove from Exposure:* Move the person to an area with fresh air immediately.
   - *Open Windows and Doors:* Ventilate the space to clear out the toxic substance.

3. **Position for Comfort:**
   - *Comfortable Position:* Help the person sit or lie down in a comfortable position.

4. **Monitor Vital Signs:**
   - *Continuous Monitoring:* Keep a close eye on the person's vital signs, including breathing and pulse. Be prepared to administer CPR if necessary.

5. **Stay with the Person:**
   - *Provide Reassurance:* Stay with the person and provide reassurance until professional medical help arrives.

Post-Inhaled Poisoning Considerations:

1. **Medical Follow-up:**
   - *Seek Urgent Medical Evaluation:* Even if initial symptoms subside, seek urgent medical evaluation to ensure comprehensive assessment and appropriate treatment.

2. **Reporting:**
   - *Provide Information:* Report the incident to relevant authorities if necessary.

3. **Preventive Measures:**
   - *Prevent Future Exposure:* Take measures to prevent future exposure to the toxic substance, and ensure proper ventilation in enclosed spaces.

In cases of inhaled poisoning, a rapid and informed response is crucial. The Basic First Aid Pocket Guide underscores the importance of calling emergency services immediately, providing fresh air, and seeking professional medical evaluation for comprehensive care.

CONTACT WITH POISONOUS SUBSTANCES

Contact with poisonous substances can occur through skin exposure. The Basic First Aid Pocket Guide outlines the following steps for recognizing and responding to contact with poisonous substances:

Recognizing Signs of Contact Poisoning:

1. **Skin Irritation:**
   - *Rashes or Burns:* Immediate skin irritation, redness, or burns.
   - *Itching or Discomfort:* Persistent itching or discomfort on the skin.

2. **Eye Irritation:**
   - *Redness:* Red or bloodshot eyes.
   - *Tearing:* eyes that are too wet or teary.

3. **Respiratory Distress:**
   - *Difficulty Breathing:* If the substance has volatile fumes, difficulty breathing may occur.

4. **General Symptoms:**
   - *Nausea or Vomiting:* Ingestion of the substance through contact may lead to nausea or vomiting.
   - *Dizziness or Weakness:* Sudden weakness or lightheadedness.

Immediate Response to Contact with Poisonous Substances:

1. **Call Emergency Services:**
   - *Urgent Action:* Call emergency services immediately. Provide information about the suspected poison and follow their guidance.

2. **Remove Contaminated Clothing:**
   - *Protective Measures:* If the substance is on clothing, remove it to prevent further exposure.
   - *Wear Gloves:* Use gloves if available to avoid direct skin contact.

3. **Rinse with Water:**
   - *Flush Affected Area:* Rinse the affected skin or eyes with copious amounts of water for at least 15 minutes.
   - *Use Eyewash Station:* If available, use an eyewash station for eye exposure.

4. **Do Not Use Chemical Neutralizers:**
   - *Avoid Neutralizing Agents:* Do not use chemical neutralizers unless advised by poison control or medical professionals.

5. **Seek Shelter from Fumes:**
   - *Move to Fresh Air:* If fumes are present, move to an area with fresh air to avoid inhalation.

6. **Monitor Vital Signs:**
   - *Continuous Monitoring:* Keep a close eye on the person's vital signs, including breathing and pulse. Be prepared to perform CPR if necessary.

7. **Stay with the Person:**
   - *Provide Reassurance:* Stay with the person and provide reassurance until professional medical help arrives.

Post-Contact Poisoning Considerations:

1. **Medical Follow-up:**
   - *Seek Urgent Medical Evaluation:* Even if initial symptoms subside, seek urgent medical evaluation to ensure comprehensive assessment and appropriate treatment.

2. **Reporting:**
   - *Provide Information:* Report the incident to relevant authorities if necessary.

3. **Preventive Measures:**
   - *Prevent Future Exposure:* Take measures to prevent future contact with the toxic substance, and use personal protective equipment when handling hazardous materials.

In cases of contact with poisonous substances, quick and appropriate action is essential. The Basic First Aid Pocket Guide emphasizes the importance of calling emergency services immediately, rinsing affected areas, and seeking professional medical evaluation for comprehensive care.

CHAPTER ELEVEN

HYPOTHERMIA AND HYPERTHERMIA

Both hypothermia and hyperthermia involve abnormal body temperature regulation and require swift attention. The Basic First Aid Pocket Guide outlines the following steps for recognizing and responding to these conditions:

Recognizing Signs of Hypothermia:

1. **Shivering:**
   - *Early Symptom:* Shivering is an initial response to cold temperatures.

2. **Confusion or Slurred Speech:**
   - *Cognitive Impairment:* Confusion, drowsiness, or slurred speech may indicate worsening hypothermia.

3. **Weak Pulse and Shallow Breathing:**
   - *Circulatory and Respiratory Issues:* As hypothermia progresses, the pulse weakens, and breathing becomes shallow.

4. **Loss of Coordination:**
   - *Difficulty Moving:* Loss of coordination and difficulty moving are advanced signs.

5. **Unconsciousness:**
   - *Severe Hypothermia:* In severe cases, the person may lose consciousness.

Immediate Response to Hypothermia:

1. **Move to Warm Environment:**
   - *Avoid Further Exposure:* Move the person to a warm environment to prevent further heat loss.
   - *Protect from Wind:* Use a barrier to shield from wind if outdoors.

2. **Remove Wet Clothing:**
   - *Promote Dryness:* Remove wet clothing and replace with dry, warm layers.
   - *Use Blankets:* Wrap the person in blankets or warm clothing.

3. **Provide Warm Drinks:**
   - *Warm, Non-Alcoholic Drinks:* Offer warm, non-alcoholic beverages to help raise body temperature.

4. **Use Warm Compresses:**
   - *Apply to Key Areas:* Apply warm compresses to the neck, chest, and groin areas.

5. **Seek Medical Attention:**
   - *Professional Evaluation:* If the person's condition is severe or not improving, seek professional medical assistance.

Recognizing Signs of Hyperthermia:

1. **High Body Temperature:**
   - *Core Temperature Above 104°F (40°C):*
Hyperthermia involves an elevated body
temperature.

2. **Hot, Dry Skin:**
   - *Lack of Sweating:* In some cases, the skin
may be hot and dry due to reduced or absent
sweating.

3. **Rapid Pulse:**
   - *Increased Heart Rate:* The heart rate may
become significantly elevated.

4. **Confusion or Dizziness:**
   - *Cognitive Impairment:* Confusion, dizziness, or
even fainting may occur.

5. **Nausea and Vomiting:**
   - *Gastrointestinal Distress:* Nausea and
vomiting may be present.

Immediate Response to Hyperthermia:

1. **Move to Cool Environment:**
   - *Avoid Further Heat Exposure:* Move the
person to a cooler environment.
   - *Use Shade or Shelter:* Provide shade or
shelter if outdoors.

2. **Cooling Measures:**
   - *Cool Compresses:* Apply cool compresses to the forehead, neck, and armpits.
   - *Use Fans or Air Conditioning:* If available, use fans or air conditioning to aid cooling.

3. **Hydration:**
   - *Encourage Fluid Intake:* Ensure the person drinks water or other hydrating fluids.
   - *Avoid Caffeine and Alcohol:* Discourage consumption of caffeine and alcohol, as they can contribute to dehydration.

4. **Loosen Clothing:**
   - *Promote Airflow:* Loosen or remove excess clothing to enhance ventilation.

5. **Seek Medical Attention:**
   - *Professional Evaluation:* If the person's condition is severe or not improving, seek professional medical assistance.

In cases of both hypothermia and hyperthermia, quick and appropriate action is crucial. The Basic First Aid Pocket Guide emphasizes the importance of recognizing signs, providing immediate care, and seeking professional medical evaluation for comprehensive management.

FROSTBITE AND COLD-RELATED INJURIES

Cold-related injuries, such as frostbite, can occur when the skin and underlying tissues freeze due to exposure to extreme cold. The Basic First Aid Pocket Guide outlines the following steps for recognizing and responding to frostbite and other cold-related injuries:

Recognizing Signs of Frostbite:

1. **Numbness or Tingling:**
   - *Early Warning:* Numbness or tingling in the affected area may be an early sign.

2. **Skin Discoloration:**
   - *Pale or White:* The skin may appear pale, white, or even bluish in color.

3. **Hardened or Waxy Skin:**
   - *Loss of Softness:* The affected skin may feel hardened or waxy to the touch.

4. **Joint or Muscle Stiffness:**
   - *Reduced Mobility:* Stiffness in joints or muscles near the frostbitten area.

5. **Severe Frostbite:**
   - *Blisters or Blackened Skin:* In severe cases, blisters or blackened skin may develop.

Immediate Response to Frostbite:

1. **Move to Warm Environment:**
   - *Avoid Further Exposure:* Move the person to a warm environment to prevent additional frostbite.
   - *Use Body Heat:* Encourage the person to use body heat from unaffected areas to warm the frostbitten parts.

2. **Remove Wet Clothing:**
   - *Promote Dryness:* Remove wet clothing and replace with dry, warm layers.
   - *Use Blankets:* Wrap the person in blankets or warm clothing.

3. **Warm Water Soak:**
   - *Submerge in Warm Water:* Immerse the affected area in warm (not hot) water for 20-30 minutes.
   - *Avoid Rubbing:* Do not rub the frostbitten area, as it can cause further damage.

4. **Avoid Rewarming if Refreezing May Occur:**
   - *Professional Guidance:* If there's a risk of refreezing, avoid rewarming until reaching professional medical assistance.

5. **Seek Medical Attention:**
   - *Professional Evaluation:* Seek professional medical attention for all cases of frostbite to assess severity and guide further treatment.

Recognizing Signs of Cold-Related Injuries (Hypothermia):

1. **Shivering:**
   - *Early Symptom:* Shivering is an initial response to cold temperatures.

2. **Confusion or Slurred Speech:**
   - *Cognitive Impairment:* Confusion, drowsiness, or slurred speech may indicate worsening hypothermia.

3. **Weak Pulse and Shallow Breathing:**
   - *Circulatory and Respiratory Issues:* As hypothermia progresses, the pulse weakens, and breathing becomes shallow.

4. **Loss of Coordination:**
   - *Difficulty Moving:* Loss of coordination and difficulty moving are advanced signs.

5. **Unconsciousness:**
   - *Severe Hypothermia:* In severe cases, the person may lose consciousness.

Immediate Response to Cold-Related Injuries (Hypothermia):

1. **Move to Warm Environment:**
   - *Avoid Further Exposure:* Move the person to a warm environment to prevent further heat loss.

- *Protect from Wind:* Use a barrier to shield from wind if outdoors.

2. **Remove Wet Clothing:**
   - *Promote Dryness:* Remove wet clothing and replace with dry, warm layers.
   - *Use Blankets:* Wrap the person in blankets or warm clothing.

3. **Provide Warm Drinks:**
   - *Warm, Non-Alcoholic Drinks:* Offer warm, non-alcoholic beverages to help raise body temperature.

4. **Use Warm Compresses:**
   - *Apply to Key Areas:* Apply warm compresses to the neck, chest, and groin areas.

5. **Seek Medical Attention:**
   - *Professional Evaluation:* If the person's condition is severe or not improving, seek professional medical assistance.

In cases of frostbite and cold-related injuries, quick and appropriate action is crucial. The Basic First Aid Pocket Guide emphasizes the importance of recognizing signs, providing immediate care, and seeking professional medical evaluation for comprehensive management.

HEAT EXHAUSTION AND HEAT STROKE

Both heat exhaustion and heat stroke are serious conditions caused by prolonged exposure to high temperatures. The Basic First Aid Pocket Guide outlines the following steps for recognizing and responding to these heat-related conditions:

Recognizing Signs of Heat Exhaustion:

1. **Heavy Sweating:**
   - *Profuse Sweating:* Excessive sweating is a common early sign of heat exhaustion.

2. **Weakness or Fatigue:**
   - *Feeling Weak:* A sense of weakness or fatigue may set in.

3. **Dizziness or Lightheadedness:**
   - *Feeling Dizzy:* Dizziness or lightheadedness may occur.

4. **Nausea or Vomiting:**
   - *Gastrointestinal Distress:* Nausea and vomiting are possible symptoms.

5. **Cool, Moist Skin:**
   - *Clammy Skin:* Skin may feel cool and moist.

Immediate Response to Heat Exhaustion:

1. **Move to a Cooler Environment:**
   - *Avoid Further Heat Exposure:* Move the person to a cooler environment to prevent worsening of symptoms.
   - *Use Shade or Shelter:* Provide shade or shelter if outdoors.

2. **Hydrate:**
   - *Encourage Fluid Intake:* Ensure the person drinks water or sports drinks to rehydrate.
   - *Avoid Caffeine and Alcohol:* Discourage consumption of caffeine and alcohol, as they can contribute to dehydration.

3. **Loosen Clothing:**
   - *Promote Airflow:* Loosen or remove excess clothing to enhance ventilation.

4. **Cooling Measures:**
   - *Use Cool Compresses:* Apply cool compresses to the forehead, neck, and armpits.
   - *Use Fans or Air Conditioning:* If available, use fans or air conditioning to aid cooling.

5. **Monitor Vital Signs:**
   - *Continuous Monitoring:* Keep a close eye on the person's vital signs, including breathing and pulse.

6. **Seek Medical Attention:**
   - *Professional Evaluation:* If symptoms persist or worsen, seek professional medical assistance.

Recognizing Signs of Heat Stroke:

1. **High Body Temperature:**
   - *Core Temperature Above 104°F (40°C):* Heat stroke involves an extremely elevated body temperature.

2. **Altered Mental State:**
   - *Confusion or Agitation:* Confusion, agitation, or even unconsciousness may occur.

3. **Dry, Hot Skin:**
   - *Lack of Sweating:* In some cases, the skin may be hot and dry due to reduced or absent sweating.

4. **Rapid Pulse:**
   - *Increased Heart Rate:* The heart rate may become significantly elevated.

5. **Nausea or Vomiting:**
   - *Gastrointestinal Distress:* Nausea and vomiting may be present.

Immediate Response to Heat Stroke:

1. **Call Emergency Services:**
   - *Urgent Action:* Call emergency services immediately. Heat stroke is a medical emergency.

2. **Move to a Cooler Environment:**

- *Avoid Further Heat Exposure:* Move the person to a cooler environment.
   - *Use Shade or Shelter:* Provide shade or shelter if outdoors.

3. **Cool the Body:**
   - *Use Cool Compresses:* Apply cool compresses to the forehead, neck, and armpits.
   - *Immerse in Cold Water:* If possible, immerse the person in cold water or use a cold shower.

4. **Hydrate:**
   - *Encourage Fluid Intake:* If conscious and able to swallow, provide cool fluids for rehydration.

5. **Monitor Vital Signs:**
   - *Continuous Monitoring:* Keep a close eye on the person's vital signs, including breathing and pulse.
   - *Start CPR if Necessary:* If the person is unconscious and not breathing, start CPR.

6. **Seek Medical Attention:**
   - *Professional Evaluation:* Even if initial measures are effective, seek professional medical assistance for comprehensive evaluation and treatment.

In cases of heat exhaustion and heat stroke, rapid and appropriate action is crucial. The Basic First Aid Pocket Guide emphasizes the importance of recognizing signs, providing immediate care, and seeking professional medical evaluation for comprehensive management.

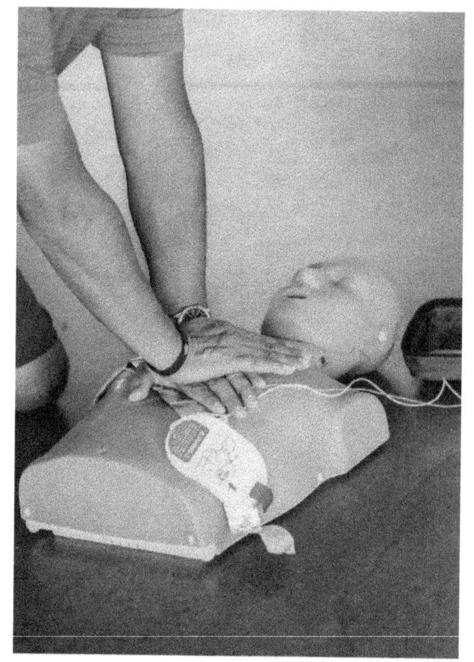

CPR

CHAPTER TWELVE

INSECTS BITES AND STINGS

Insect bites and stings are common occurrences, and while most are harmless, some can cause allergic reactions or transmit diseases. The Basic First Aid Pocket Guide outlines the following steps for recognizing and responding to insect bites and stings:

Recognizing Signs of Insect Bites and Stings:

1. **Redness and Swelling:**
   - *Localized Reaction:* Redness and swelling around the bite or sting site are common.

2. **Itching or Pain:**
   - *Mild Discomfort:* Itching or pain may be experienced, varying in intensity.

3. **Raised Skin:**
   - *Hive-like Reaction:* Raised, hive-like bumps may develop.

4. **Localized Heat:**
   - *Warmth Around Site:* The affected area may feel warm to the touch.

5. **Inflammation:**
   - *Inflammatory Response:* Inflammation is a typical reaction.

Immediate Response to Insect Bites and Stings:

1. **Remove Stinger if Present:**
   - *Scrape or Pinch:* Use a flat-edged object to gently scrape away the stinger or pinch it out if visible.
   - *Avoid Squeezing:* Do not use tweezers or fingers to squeeze the stinger, as it may release more venom.

2. **Clean the Area:**
   - *Mild Soap and Water:* Clean the bite or sting site with mild soap and water to reduce the risk of infection.

3. **Apply Cold Compress:**
   - *Reduce Swelling:* Apply a cold compress or ice pack wrapped in a cloth to reduce swelling and ease discomfort.

4. **Use Over-the-Counter Creams:**
   - *Antihistamine or Hydrocortisone Cream:* Apply over-the-counter creams to alleviate itching or swelling.
   - *Avoid Scratching:* Discourage scratching to prevent infection and further irritation.

5. **Elevate if Possible:**
   - *Reduce Swelling:* If the bite or sting is on a limb, elevate it to reduce swelling.

6. **Take Pain Relievers:**
   - *Non-prescription Pain Relievers:* Consider non-prescription pain relievers like ibuprofen or acetaminophen if needed.

7. **Monitor for Allergic Reactions:**
   - *Watch for Severe Symptoms:* Keep an eye for signs of severe allergic reactions, such as difficulty breathing, swelling of the face or throat, and a rapid or weak pulse.

8. **Seek Medical Attention:**
   - *Allergic Reactions:* If the person experiences severe allergic reactions or if the bite/sting is from a venomous creature, seek medical attention promptly.

Preventive Measures:

1. **Avoiding Insect Exposure:**
   - *Use Repellent:* Apply insect repellent with DEET or other recommended ingredients.
   - *Wear Protective Clothing:* Wear long sleeves, pants, and closed shoes in areas prone to insect bites.

2. **Preventing Allergic Reactions:**

- *Carry an EpiPen:* Individuals with known severe allergies should carry an epinephrine auto-injector (EpiPen) as prescribed.

3. **Understanding Local Wildlife:**
   - *Awareness:* Be aware of local insects and wildlife to minimize encounters with venomous species.

Insect bites and stings are generally manageable with basic first aid, but severe reactions require immediate medical attention. The Basic First Aid Pocket Guide emphasizes prompt care, monitoring for allergic reactions, and seeking professional help when necessary.

BEE STINGS

Bee stings can cause discomfort and, in some cases, allergic reactions. The Basic First Aid Pocket Guide outlines the following steps for recognizing and responding to bee stings:

Recognizing Signs of Bee Stings:

1. **Immediate Pain:**
   - *Sharp or Burning Pain:* Immediate pain at the sting site.

2. **Redness and Swelling:**

   - *Localized Reaction:* Redness and swelling
around the sting area.

3. **Itching or Discomfort:**
   - *Mild to Moderate Itching:* Itching or discomfort
may follow the initial pain.

4. **Raised Skin:**
   - *Hive-like Reaction:* Raised, hive-like bumps
may develop.

5. **Possibly a Stinger Left Behind:**
   - *Visible Stinger:* In some cases, the bee's
stinger may be left behind in the skin.

Immediate Response to Bee Stings:

1. **Remove Stinger if Present:**
   - *Scrape or Pinch:* Use a flat-edged object to
gently scrape away the stinger or pinch it out if
visible.
   - *Avoid Squeezing:* Do not use tweezers or
fingers to squeeze the stinger, as it may release
more venom.

2. **Clean the Area:**
   - *Mild Soap and Water:* Clean the sting site with
mild soap and water to reduce the risk of infection.

3. **Apply Cold Compress:**

- *Reduce Swelling:* Apply a cold compress or ice pack wrapped in a cloth to reduce swelling and ease discomfort.

4. **Use Over-the-Counter Creams:**
   - *Antihistamine or Hydrocortisone Cream:* Apply over-the-counter creams to alleviate itching or swelling.
   - *Avoid Scratching:* Discourage scratching to prevent infection and further irritation.

5. **Elevate if Possible:**
   - *Reduce Swelling:* If the sting is on a limb, elevate it to reduce swelling.

6. **Take Pain Relievers:**
   - *Non-prescription Pain Relievers:* Consider non-prescription pain relievers like ibuprofen or acetaminophen if needed.

7. **Monitor for Allergic Reactions:**
   - *Watch for Severe Symptoms:* Keep an eye for signs of severe allergic reactions, such as difficulty breathing, swelling of the face or throat, and a rapid or weak pulse.

8. **Seek Medical Attention:**
   - *Allergic Reactions:* If the person experiences severe allergic reactions or if stung multiple times, seek medical attention promptly.

Preventive Measures:

1. **Avoiding Bee Stings:**
   - *Stay Calm and Still:* If a bee is near, stay calm and still. Rapid movements may provoke an attack.
   - *Avoid Fragrances:* Bees are attracted to sweet scents, so avoid wearing strong fragrances.

2. **Wearing Protective Clothing:**
   - *Cover Exposed Skin:* When in areas with bees, wear long sleeves, pants, and closed shoes.
   - *Avoid Bright Colors:* Bees are attracted to bright colors, so consider wearing neutral tones.

3. **Understanding Bee Behavior:**
   - *Awareness:* Be aware of bee nests or hives in the surroundings and avoid disturbing them.

Bee stings are generally manageable with basic first aid, but severe reactions require immediate medical attention. The Basic First Aid Pocket Guide emphasizes prompt care, monitoring for allergic reactions, and seeking professional help when necessary.

TICK BITES

Tick bites can lead to potential health concerns, including the risk of tick-borne diseases. The Basic First Aid Pocket Guide outlines the following steps for recognizing and responding to tick bites:

Recognizing Signs of Tick Bites:

1. **Presence of a Tick:**
   - *Visible Tick:* The presence of a tick attached to the skin.

2. **Redness and Swelling:**
   - *Localized Reaction:* Redness and swelling around the bite site.

3. **Itching or Discomfort:**
   - *Mild to Moderate Itching:* Itching or discomfort in the area of the tick bite.

4. **Possibly a Raised Area:**
   - *Papular Reaction:* In some cases, a raised area or a small bump may develop.

5. **Site of Attachment:**
   - *Central Point of Attachment:* The tick may be centrally attached to the skin.

Immediate Response to Tick Bites:

1. **Safely Remove the Tick:**
   - *Use Fine-Tipped Tweezers:* Using fine-tipped tweezers, grasp the tick as close to the skin's surface as you can.
   - *Avoid Crushing the Tick:* Pull upward with steady, even pressure. Avoid twisting or crushing the tick.

2. **Clean the Bite Area:**
   - *Mild Soap and Water:* Clean the bite area with mild soap and water after tick removal.

3. **Apply Antiseptic:**
   - *Antiseptic Ointment:* Apply an antiseptic ointment to the bite site to reduce the risk of infection.

4. **Monitor for Signs of Infection:**
   - *Watch for Redness or Swelling:* Keep an eye on the bite area for any signs of infection, such as increasing redness or swelling.

5. **Save the Tick:**
   - *Preserve Evidence:* If possible, save the tick in a sealed container for identification in case of later complications.

6. **Seek Medical Attention:**
   - *Fever or Rash:* If the person develops fever or a rash after a tick bite, seek medical attention promptly.

Preventive Measures:

1. **Avoiding Tick Exposure:**
   - *Wear Protective Clothing:* When in areas with ticks, wear long sleeves, pants, and closed shoes.
   - *Use Tick Repellent:* Apply insect repellent with DEET or other recommended ingredients.

2. **Checking for Ticks:**
   - *Perform Tick Checks:* After spending time outdoors, perform thorough tick checks on yourself, family members, and pets.
   - *Shower After Outdoor Activities:* Showering can help wash off ticks that have not yet attached.

3. **Creating Tick-Safe Environments:**
   - *Clear Vegetation:* Keep grass short and clear vegetation around homes to reduce tick habitats.
   - *Use Tick Control Products:* Consider using tick control products on pets and treating outdoor areas.

4. **Being Aware of Tick-Borne Diseases:**
   - *Know Local Risks:* Be aware of the prevalence of tick-borne diseases in your local area.
   - *Seek Prompt Treatment:* If symptoms of tick-borne illnesses, such as Lyme disease, arise, seek medical attention promptly.

Tick bites should be addressed promptly to reduce the risk of complications. The Basic First Aid Pocket Guide emphasizes the importance of safe tick removal, thorough cleaning, and monitoring for any signs of infection or tick-borne diseases. If concerns arise, seeking medical attention is crucial.

SPIDER BITES

Spider bites can cause various reactions, ranging from mild irritation to severe symptoms. The Basic First Aid Pocket Guide outlines the following steps for recognizing and responding to spider bites:

Recognizing Signs of Spider Bites:

1. **Immediate Pain or Sting:**
   - *Sharp or Burning Pain:* Immediate pain or a stinging sensation at the bite site.

2. **Redness and Swelling:**
   - *Localized Reaction:* Redness and swelling around the bite site are common.

3. **Itching or Discomfort:**
   - *Mild to Moderate Itching:* Itching or discomfort in the area of the spider bite.

4. **Possibly a Raised Area:**
   - *Papular Reaction:* In some cases, a raised area or a small bump may develop.

5. **Central Ulcer or Blister:**
   - *Ulcer or Blister Formation:* Some spider bites may result in the formation of a central ulcer or blister.

Immediate Response to Spider Bites:

1. **Clean the Bite Area:**
   - *Mild Soap and Water:* Clean the bite area with mild soap and water to reduce the risk of infection.

2. **Apply Antiseptic:**
   - *Antiseptic Ointment:* Apply an antiseptic ointment to the bite site to reduce the risk of infection.

3. **Use Cold Compress:**
   - *Reduce Swelling:* Apply a cold compress or ice pack wrapped in a cloth to reduce swelling and ease discomfort.

4. **Take Pain Relievers:**
   - *Non-prescription Pain Relievers:* Consider non-prescription pain relievers like ibuprofen or acetaminophen if needed.

5. **Avoid Scratching:**
   - *Prevent Infection:* Discourage scratching to prevent infection and further irritation.

6. **Elevate if Possible:**
   - *Reduce Swelling:* If the bite is on a limb, elevate it to reduce swelling.

7. **Monitor for Signs of Infection:**
   - *Watch for Redness or Swelling:* Keep an eye on the bite area for any signs of infection, such as increasing redness or swelling.

8. **Seek Medical Attention:**
   - *Severe Symptoms:* If the person experiences severe symptoms, such as difficulty breathing, chest pain, or systemic reactions, seek medical attention promptly.

Preventive Measures:

1. **Avoiding Spider Bites:**
   - *Shake Out Clothing:* Before putting on clothing that has been stored, shake it out to dislodge any spiders.
   - *Check Shoes and Bedding:* Regularly inspect shoes and bedding for spiders before use.

2. **Creating Spider-Resistant Environments:**
   - *Seal Cracks and Crevices:* Seal cracks and crevices in homes to reduce spider entry points.
   - *Keep Outdoor Areas Clear:* Clear debris and clutter around homes to reduce spider habitats.

3. **Being Aware of Venomous Spiders:**
   - *Know Local Species:* Be aware of venomous spiders in your local area and take appropriate precautions.

Spider bites are usually mild and can be managed with basic first aid. However, if severe symptoms occur or if the bite is from a potentially dangerous spider, seeking medical attention is crucial. The Basic First Aid Pocket Guide emphasizes prompt care, monitoring for signs of infection or severe reactions, and seeking professional help when necessary.

CHAPTER THIRTEEN

BASIC FIRST AID KIT ESSENTIALS

Having a well-equipped first aid kit is essential for handling minor injuries and emergencies. The Basic First Aid Pocket Guide outlines the following essentials for a basic first aid kit:

1. **Adhesive Bandages:**
   - *Various Sizes:* Include a variety of adhesive bandages to cover different wound sizes.

2. **Sterile Gauze Pads:**
   - *Different Sizes:* Sterile gauze pads for wound dressing and covering.

3. **Adhesive Tape:**
   - *Securing Dressings:* A roll of adhesive tape to secure bandages and dressings.

4. **Antiseptic Wipes or Solution:**
   - *Cleaning Wounds:* Antiseptic wipes or solution for cleaning cuts and abrasions.

5. **Scissors:**
   - *Cutting Materials:* A pair of scissors for cutting tape, gauze, or clothing.

6. **Tweezers:**
   - *Removing Splinters or Ticks:* Tweezers for safely removing splinters or ticks.

7. **Disposable Gloves:**
   - *Protective Barrier:* Disposable gloves to protect against bodily fluids during first aid.

8. **Instant Cold Compress:**
   - *Reducing Swelling:* An instant cold compress for treating injuries that involve swelling.

9. **Pain Relievers:**
   - *Non-prescription Medication:* Over-the-counter pain relievers like acetaminophen or ibuprofen.

10. **First Aid Manual:**
    - *Guidance and Reference:* A basic first aid manual providing guidance on common injuries and emergencies.

11. **CPR Face Shield:**
    - *Protective Barrier for CPR:* A CPR face shield for providing protection during mouth-to-mouth resuscitation.

12. **Emergency Blanket:**
    - *Heat Retention:* An emergency blanket for warmth and protection against hypothermia.

13. **Burn Cream or Gel:**

  - *Treating Minor Burns:* Burn cream or gel for soothing and treating minor burns.

14. **Elastic Bandage:**
   - *Supporting Sprains:* An elastic bandage for providing support to sprained joints.

15. **Triangular Bandage:**
   - *Sling or Tourniquet:* A triangular bandage that can be used as a sling or tourniquet.

16. **Cotton Swabs and Cotton Balls:**
   - *Applying Ointments:* Cotton swabs and balls for applying ointments or cleaning.

17. **Antihistamine Tablets:**
   - *Allergic Reactions:* Antihistamine tablets for treating mild allergic reactions.

18. **Pencil and Notepad:**
   - *Recording Information:* A pencil and notepad for recording important information.

19. **Hydrocortisone Cream:**
   - *Skin Irritations:* Hydrocortisone cream for alleviating itching and skin irritations.

20. **Personal Medications:**
   - *Individual Needs:* Any necessary personal medications or prescription items.

Regularly check and replenish your first aid kit to ensure that supplies are up-to-date and available when needed. Additionally, consider including any specific items tailored to your family's medical needs or activities. Always seek professional medical assistance for severe injuries or emergencies. The Basic First Aid Pocket Guide emphasizes the importance of being prepared and having the necessary tools to respond effectively in various situations.

CONCLUSION

In the realm of health and safety, being equipped with basic first aid knowledge and essentials is a fundamental aspect of preparedness. The Basic First Aid Pocket Guide serves as a valuable resource, providing quick and concise information to empower individuals in handling common injuries and emergencies.

From understanding the ABCs of first aid, including assessing the scene and calling for help, to comprehensive guidance on CPR, addressing injuries, and managing various medical situations, this pocket guide aims to be a companion for individuals seeking practical insights into immediate care.

By emphasizing preventive measures, recognizing signs of emergencies, and offering step-by-step responses, the guide strives to instill confidence in individuals to act swiftly and effectively during critical moments. The integration of key topics, ranging from insect bites to heat-related conditions, underscores the guide's versatility in addressing a spectrum of health concerns.

Moreover, the inclusion of essential items for a first aid kit reinforces the importance of preparation. A well-equipped kit can make a significant difference in providing timely assistance during unforeseen events.

In conclusion, the Basic First Aid Pocket Guide serves as a valuable tool, promoting a proactive approach to health and safety. By fostering a culture of preparedness, individuals can play a vital role in creating safer environments for themselves and those around them. Remember, while the guide offers valuable insights, seeking professional medical assistance remains paramount in cases of severe injuries or emergencies. Stay informed, stay prepared, and prioritize safety in every situation.